A Practical Approach to
Cervical Cancer Screening Techniques

A Practical Approach to Cervical Cancer Screening Techniques

T Radha Bai Prabhu

MD DGO MNAMS FRCOG FRCS PhD

Professor
Department of Obstetrics and Gynecology
Meenakshi Medical College and Research Institute
Kancheepuram, Tamil Nadu, India

Formerly Director and Superintendent
Institute of Obstetrics and Gynecology
Government Hospital for Women and Children
Chennai, Tamil Nadu, India

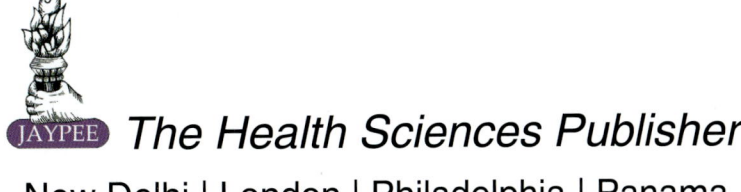

The Health Sciences Publisher

New Delhi | London | Philadelphia | Panama

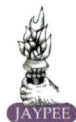 **Jaypee Brothers Medical Publishers (P) Ltd**

Headquarters

Jaypee Brothers Medical Publishers (P) Ltd
4838/24, Ansari Road, Daryaganj
New Delhi 110 002, India
Phone: +91-11-43574357
Fax: +91-11-43574314
Email: jaypee@jaypeebrothers.com

Overseas Offices

J.P. Medical Ltd
83 Victoria Street, London
SW1H 0HW (UK)
Phone: +44 20 3170 8910
Fax: +44 (0)20 3008 6180
Email: info@jpmedpub.com

Jaypee-Highlights Medical Publishers Inc
City of Knowledge, Bld. 237, Clayton
Panama City, Panama
Phone: +1 507-301-0496
Fax: +1 507-301-0499
Email: cservice@jphmedical.com

Jaypee Medical Inc
The Bourse
111 South Independence Mall East
Suite 835, Philadelphia, PA 19106, USA
Phone: +1 267-519-9789
Email: jpmed.us@gmail.com

Jaypee Brothers Medical Publishers (P) Ltd
17/1-B Babar Road, Block-B, Shaymali
Mohammadpur, Dhaka-1207
Bangladesh
Mobile: +08801912003485
Email: jaypeedhaka@gmail.com

Jaypee Brothers Medical Publishers (P) Ltd
Bhotahity, Kathmandu, Nepal
Phone: +977-9741283608
Email: kathmandu@jaypeebrothers.com

Website: www.jaypeebrothers.com
Website: www.jaypeedigital.com

© 2015, Jaypee Brothers Medical Publishers

The views and opinions expressed in this book are solely those of the original contributor(s)/author(s) and do not necessarily represent those of editor(s) of the book.

All rights reserved. No part of this publication may be reproduced, stored or transmitted in any form or by any means, electronic, mechanical, photocopying, recording or otherwise, without the prior permission in writing of the publishers.

All brand names and product names used in this book are trade names, service marks, trademarks or registered trademarks of their respective owners. The publisher is not associated with any product or vendor mentioned in this book.

Medical knowledge and practice change constantly. This book is designed to provide accurate, authoritative information about the subject matter in question. However, readers are advised to check the most current information available on procedures included and check information from the manufacturer of each product to be administered, to verify the recommended dose, formula, method and duration of administration, adverse effects and contraindications. It is the responsibility of the practitioner to take all appropriate safety precautions. Neither the publisher nor the author(s)/editor(s) assume any liability for any injury and/or damage to persons or property arising from or related to use of material in this book.

This book is sold on the understanding that the publisher is not engaged in providing professional medical services. If such advice or services are required, the services of a competent medical professional should be sought.

Every effort has been made where necessary to contact holders of copyright to obtain permission to reproduce copyright material. If any have been inadvertently overlooked, the publisher will be pleased to make the necessary arrangements at the first opportunity.

Inquiries for bulk sales may be solicited at: jaypee@jaypeebrothers.com

A Practical Approach to Cervical Cancer Screening Techniques

First Edition: **2015**

ISBN 978-93-5152-469-4

Printed at : Samrat Offset Pvt. Ltd.

Dedicated to

My Mother, Mrs T Rajarathinam

Preface

Cervical cancer is both preventable and curable provided it is detected in its pre-invasive stage or in the early stage. India accounts for nearly 16% of the global burden and about 1,30,000 new cases are diagnosed per year and more than 75,000 women die of it annually.

The main aim of this book entitled *Practical Approach to Cervical Cancer Screening Techniques* is to sensitize the postgraduate trainees and practicing gynecologists in the prevention of cervical carcinoma.

My initial interest in colposcopy was stimulated by Late Professor Dr Sheila Rajarathinam at Government RSRM Lying-in Hospital, Chennai, Tamil Nadu. She sent me to Nowroji Wadia Maternity Hospital, Mumbai, Maharashtra, for my training in colposcopy in 1984. Subsequently, I was trained by Dr Magid Zaklama, Consultant, Birch Hill Hospital, UK for 3 years. Under his mentorship, my technique and interpreting skills and abilities improved, which made me an accredited Colposcopist with the British Society of Colposcopy and Cervical Pathology. I am grateful to him, for his efforts and interest shown on me to make an experienced Colposcopist.

With my years of clinical experience, I have written this book with an aim to teach the clinicians, the various techniques used in cervical cancer screening in a very simple way so that they can be incorporated in to their day-to-day clinical practice.

I hope this book will be of great value to the readers and will kindle their interest to venture into techniques to prevent cervical carcinoma.

T Radha Bai Prabhu

Contents

1. **Introduction** — 1
2. **Cervical Anatomy** — 3
   Histology 3
   The Squamous Epithelium 4
   Columnar Epithelium 4
   Shedding of Cells in Various Age Groups 5
   Cytoplasm 5
   Nuclear Pattern 6
   Exposure to Estrogen 6
   Exposure to Progestogens 6
   Childhood Period 6
   Reproductive Age 6
   Pregnancy 6
   The Squamocolumnar Junction (SCJ) 6
   Metaplastic Epithelium 6
   Blood Supply to the Cervix 7
   Nerve Supply 7
3. **Etiology and Risk Factors for Cervical Carcinoma** — 8
   Metaplasia in the Transformation Zone 8
   Exposure to Oncogen 8
   Immune Status of the Individual 9
   Smoking and Cervical Carcinoma 9
   Co-infection with Sexually Transmitted Infectious Agents and Cervical Carcinoma 9
4. **Human Papillomavirus and Cervical Carcinoma** — 10
   Oncogenesis of HPV 10
   High-risk and Low-risk-type HPVs 10
   The HPV Cell Cycle 11
5. **Pathogenesis of Cervical Carcinoma** — 12
6. **Progression and Regression of CIN Lesions** — 14
7. **Histology of Cervical Intraepithelial Neoplasia** — 15
   CIN1 lesions 15
   CIN2 Lesions 15
   CIN3 Lesions 15
   Adenocarcinoma In Situ (AIS) 16
   Histopathology of Invasive Cancers 17
8. **Screening Tests for Cervical Carcinoma** — 20
   Criteria for a Screening Test 20
   Screening Techniques for Cervical Cancer 20
   Cervical Cytology 20
   The Papanicolaou Smear 20
   The 2001 (Revised) Bethesda System of Reporting 21
   Negative for Intraepithelial Lesion or Malignancy (NIL) 21
   Epithelial Cell Abnormalities 22
   Glandular Cells 22
   Adequacy of the Specimen 22
   Sample Collection for Cervical Cytology 22
   Timing 22
   Required Supplies for Sampling 22
   Taking Pap Smear 23
   Use of Endocervical Brush 24
   Use of Plastic Broom 24
   Evaluation of Conventional Pap Smear 24
   The Major Causes of False-negative Results 25
   Inadequate Sampling 25
   Inappropriate Sample Technique 25
   Errors in Interpretation 25
   Professional Error 25
   Liquid-based Thin-layer Cytology (LBC) 25
   Method of Collecting and Processing of Sample 26
   Advantages of LBC 26
   Limitations of LBC 26
   Automated Screening Technology 27
   Papnet 27
   Efficacy of Liquid-based Cytology 27
   Frequency of Pap Smear Testing 27
   Post Hysterectomy 28
   Post Hysterectomy Smear 28
9. **HPV DNA Testing** — 29
10. **Cytology of Normal and Abnormal Cells of Cervix** — 32
    Normal Cytology 32
    Inflammatory Smear 33
    Atypical Squamous Cells of Undetermined Significance (ASC-US) 33
    Atypical Squamous Cells of Undetermined Significance Cannot Exclude HSIL 33
    The Cytology of Low-grade Squamous Intraepithelial Lesion (LSIL) 33

High-grade Squamous Intraepithelial Lesion (HSIL) *34*
Cytology of Squamous Cell Carcinoma *34*
Cytology of Cervical Adenocarcinoma *34*
Cytology Changes in Pregnancy *36*

11. Management of Abnormal Cytology Cell Results — 37
Management of Atypical Squamous Cells *37*
Management of ASC-US *37*
Management of ASC-US in Special Populations *38*
Management of Postmenopausal Women *38*
Management of Pregnant Women *38*
Management of Immunosuppressed Women *38*
Management of Women with ASC-H *39*
Management of Women with LSIL *39*
Management of Special Population with LSIL *39*
Management of High-grade Squamous Intraepithelial Lesion (HSIL) *40*
HSIL in Special Population *40*
Management of Pregnant Women with HSIL *41*
Management of Atypical Glandular Cells and Adenocarcinoma In Situ *41*
Initial Evaluation of Women with Atypical Glandular Cells (AGC)— NOS *41*
Subsequent Evaluation and Post- Colposcopy Management *41*
Evaluation of AGC in Pregnancy *42*

12. Colposcopy — 43
Indications for Colposcopy *43*
Abnormal Smear Necessitating Referral for Colposcopy *43*
Contraindication *43*
Advantages of Colposcopy *43*
Colposcopy Equipment and Method *44*
The Colposcopy Equipment *44*
Digital Video Colposcopy *45*
Maintenance *46*
Chemicals Used during Colposcopy *46*
Preparation of 5% Acetic Acid *46*
Lugol's Iodine Solution *46*
Ingredients *46*
Monsel's Solution *46*
The Reaction May Emit Heat *47*
Silver Nitrate Sticks *47*
Effect of Acetic Acid on Cervical Epithelium *47*
Effect of Lugol's Iodine on Cervical Epithelium—Schiller's Test *48*
Preoperative Evaluation and Preparation *48*
Informed Consent for Colposcopy *48*
Technique of Colposcopy *49*

13. Interpretation of Colposcopy Findings — 51
Natural History of Cervical Epithelium *51*
Original Squamocolumnar Junction *51*
Squamous Metaplasia *52*
New Squamocolumnar Junction *52*
The Transformation Zone (TZ) *52*
Tissue Basis for Colposcopy *52*
Epithelium *53*
Stroma *53*
Surface Configuration *53*
International Colposcopic Terminology *53*
Colposcopic Appearance of Tissues *53*
Normal Colposcopic Findings *54*
Vascular Pattern of Metaplastic Epithelium *55*
Abnormal Colposcopic Findings *56*
Acetowhite Epithelium *56*
Abnormal Vascular Patterns *59*
In Adenocarcinoma *61*
Schiller's Test *61*
Leukoplakia *61*
Surface Contour *63*
Line of Demarcation *63*
Location of Lesion *63*
Significance of Abnormal Colposcopic Findings in Non-neoplastic Lesions *64*
Indications for Endocervical Assessment *64*
Satisfactory and Unsatisfactory Colposcopy *65*
Satisfactory Colposcopy *65*
Unsatisfactory Colposcopy *65*
Measures to Overcome Unsatisfactory Colposcopy *66*
Documentation of Colposcopic Findings *66*
Colposcopic Grading of Lesions *66*
Coppleson's Grading of Colposcopic Findings *67*
Reid's Colposcopic Assessment System (RCI) *67*
Lesion Margin *68*
Acetowhitening *70*
Vascular Pattern *71*
Iodine Staining *72*
The RCI Clinical Correlation *73*
Simplified Reid's Colposcopic Index *74*
Reporting of Simplified RCI *74*
Colposcopy Appearance of Benign, CIN and Malignant Lesions of the Cervix *75*
Ectropion of the Cervix *75*
Colposcopic Appearance of Metaplasia *75*
Nabothian Cyst *75*
Endocervical Polyps *75*
Colposcopy Appearance in Postmenopausal Women *76*
Infection of the Cervix *77*
Colposcopy in Pregnancy *77*
Low-grade Intraepithelial Neoplasia *82*

Difficulties in Interpreting Low-grade Lesions *82*
Colposcopy Findings in High-grade Lesions *83*
Colposcopy in Invasive Cancer *86*
Colposcopy Findings in Adenocarcinoma In Situ and Adenocarcinoma *86*

14. Visual Inspection Methods (VIA and VILI)   89
Visual Screening Techniques *89*
Advantages of Visual Screening *89*
Disadvantages of Visual Screening *89*
Other Issues Related to Visual Screening *90*
Visual Inspection with Acetic Acid (VIA) *90*
Basis of VIA *90*
Effect of Acetic Acid on Various Tissues *90*
Effect of Acetic Acid on Squamous Epithelium *90*
Effect of Acetic Acid on Columnar Epithelium *90*
Effect of Acetic Acid on Other Epithelia *90*
Intensity and Duration of Whiteness *90*
Borders of the Lesion *90*
Location of the Lesion *91*
Visual Inspection with Lugol's Iodine (VILI) *91*
Procedure of VIA and VILI *91*
Informed Consent for VIA and VILI *91*
Technique of VIA and VILI *91*
Effect of Acetic Acid and Iodine on Cervical Epithelium *92*
Reporting the Results of VIA *92*
VIA Negative *92*
VIA Positive *92*
Outcome of VILI *93*
VILI Positive *94*
Invasive Cancer *94*
Treatment *95*
Efficacy of VIA and VILI *95*

15. Cell Cycle Markers   96

16. Polarprobe   97
Principle *97*
Advantages *97*

17. Laser-induced Fluorescence   98

18. Speculoscopy   99

19. Cervicography   100
Advantages *100*
Limitations *100*

20. Colposcopy Training Log Book   101
Introduction *101*
Purpose of the Log Book *101*
Modules of the Curriculum *101*
Levels of Competence in Practical Experience Section *101*
Number of Colposcopies to be Done *101*
Theoretical Understanding *101*
Normal Cervix *101*
Equipment *101*
The Colposcopy Procedure *102*
Practical Considerations *102*
Preliminary Skills *102*
Colposcopic Examination *102*
Normal Cervix *102*
Abnormal Lower Genital Tract *102*
Practical Procedures *102*
Administration *102*
Communication *103*

References   *105*
Index   *109*

Chapter 1

Introduction

Cervical cancer is increasingly recognized to be a global problem. It has a devastating effect on the lives of women worldwide, particularly those living in developing countries. According to the latest global estimates, 493,243 new cases of cervical cancer are reported every year, and 274,000 women die of the disease annually. Out of the 493,243 new cases, about 83% are reported from the developing countries[1] **(Figure 1-1)**.

The major reasons for high cervical cancer rates in developing countries are due to lack of effective screening programs, nonavailability of adequate treatment strategies for preinvasive lesions and lack of awareness among women about the available healthcare facilities to prevent cervical cancer and failure to seek such facilities to prevent cervical cancer. Highest rates of cervical cancer are reported from South America, Sub-Saharan Africa and parts of Asia. Cervical carcinoma is the most common cancer among the Indian women.[2] More than 132,000 new cases, approximately one-fourth of global total, are reported from India every year and among them, 74,118 women die due to cervical cancer.[1] Cervical cancer is both preventable and curable, provided it is detected in its preinvasive stage or in the early stage. One of the success stories in Medicine is the prevention of cervical cancer by screening programs. Despite concerns about false-negative smears, in countries that have implemented regular screening programs, the incidence of cervical carcinoma has dropped dramatically and that of the detected preinvasive lesions has risen sharply. As a result, nearly 80% of cervical cancers are detected early and cured. In a developing country like India, there is technical and economical constraint in implementing such screening programs as well as there is ignorance among women about the availability of screening methods, and lack of knowledge about the warning symptoms of cancer cervix. This precludes early detection; therefore, nearly 80% of cervical cancers are detected at stage III and above, therefore incurable.

Cervical cancer has a long preclinical course. The precancerous changes in cervical tissue can linger for many years before becoming a cervical carcinoma. This window period gives us an opportunity for screening. As the cervix is accessible for exploration and investigation, by various strategies, these precancerous lesions can be identified and, if successfully treated, these lesions will not develop into cervical carcinoma. For the screening program to be effective, population coverage should be wide and should be screened at regular intervals. The average age of diagnosis of cervical carcinoma at the Institute of Obstetrics and

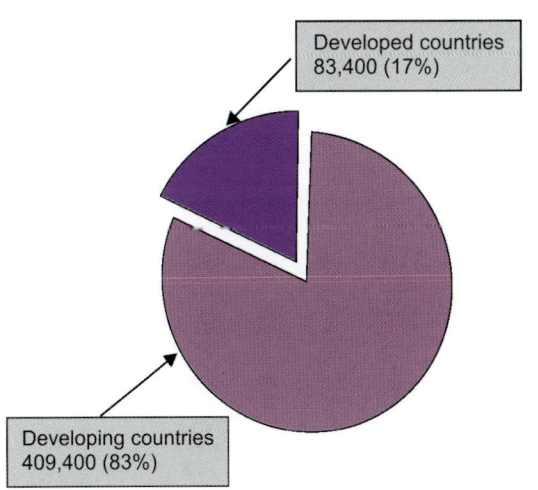

Figure 1-1: New Cervical Cancer Cases Worldwide, 2002 estimates

Gynaecology, Chennai was 50 years, 20.8% were less than 40 years, 38.4% were between 41 and 50 years and 40.8% were more than 60 years of age. There is bimodal distribution with peaks at 45–50 years and 55–60 years. The youngest patient was 30 years and the oldest was 80 years old.

The aim of cervical screening is to prevent invasive carcinoma by diagnosing and treating women with high-grade cervical lesions. There are many challenges in establishing cervical cancer screening program in developing countries. Cytological evaluation by Pap test is a simple technique to detect preinvasive stage of cervical carcinoma and has been effective in places where the coverage and quality of services are high and where Pap test can be done at regular intervals.

The major problems in organizing cytological screening in developing countries is lack of clinical expertise, trained physicians, nurses, technicians, strategies to maintain quality and interpretation of Pap smear samples, limited capacity for confirmatory testing with colposcopy and biopsy, difficulty in the follow-up of patients and facilities for treatment. In a country like India with vast population and financial constraints, most women have never had a Pap smear.

Therefore, World Health Organization (WHO), 1992 has recommended that in low resource sittings, the aim should be to screen every woman at least once in her life time between 35 and 45 years.[3,4] An Indian study has shown that one life time screening would result in reduction of 20–30% in the life time risk of cervical carcinoma.[5]

Because of the limitations and challenges in implementing cytological evaluation of cervix in developing countries, Alliance for Cervical Cancer Prevention (ACCP) has studied alternate approaches for screening, namely visual screening by VIA (Visual inspection with acetic acid) and VILI (Visual inspection with Lugol's iodine) and HPV testing.

Over the years, WHO has advocated 'down staging' by visual inspection of the cervix as a more realistic approach to active coverage in developing countries than cytology screening.[6]

The main aim of this book is to sensitize the postgraduate trainees and practicing gynecologists in preventing cervical carcinoma by detecting preinvasive lesions by screening methods. The discussion focuses on the practical approach to cervical screening techniques, describing the methodology and interpretation in detail.

Chapter 2

Cervical Anatomy

To understand the various screening approaches used in the detection of precancerous lesions of the cervix, it is important that one has a good knowledge about the anatomy of the cervix. Depending upon the age, parity and the hormonal status of the woman, the size and shape of the cervix varies. In nulliparous women, the cervix appears small and the external os is a small circular opening. In multiparous women, who have delivered by the vaginal route, the cervix is bulky and the external os is wide and gaping and appears as a transverse slit. Occasionally, there is marked eversion of the ectocervix due to torn cervix. In pregnancy, the cervix appears hypertrophied and patulous. Often there is marked ectopy of the cervix **(Figure 2-1)**.

In postmenopausal women, the cervix is atrophic and button-like or may be flushed with the vagina **(Figure 2-2)**. The above knowledge will help the clinician is choosing the appropriate technique for screening.

HISTOLOGY

The cervical tissue has a stromal layer over which epithelial cells are arranged. The stroma of the cervix is composed of vessels, lymphatics and nerve supply to the cervix. The epithelial cells of the cervix are squamous epithelium, which covers the ectocervix and the columnar epithelium, which lines the endocervical canal. The point at which the

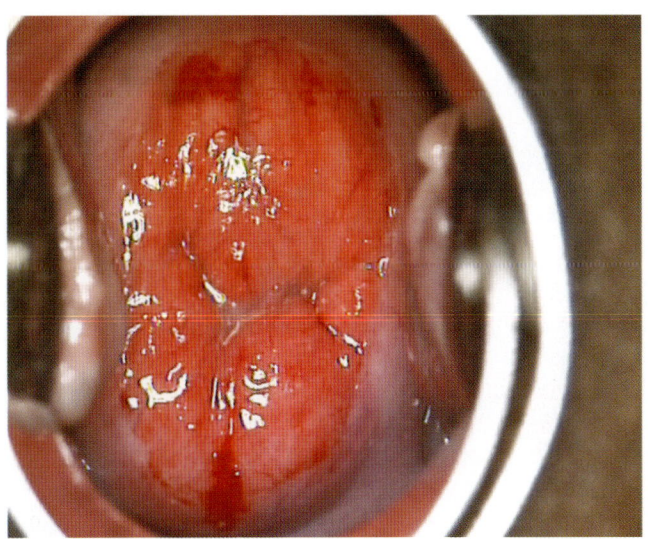

Figure 2-1: Ectopy of the cervix in pregnancy

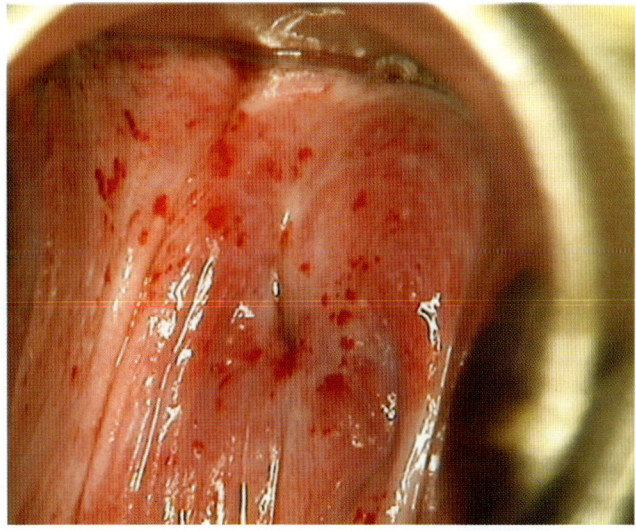

Figure 2-2: Postmenopausal cervix—atrophic, thin, flushed with the vault and brittle with petechial hemorrhages

squamous and columnar epithelium meet is called squamocolumnar junction (SCJ).

THE SQUAMOUS EPITHELIUM

The squamous epithelium of the ectocervix is multilayered, non-keratinizing and contains glycogen. The epithelial cell layer does not have blood vessels. Because of the multiple layer, it does not transmit the color from the underlying blood vessels. Therefore, on naked-eye inspection, the surface of the ectocervix appears opaque and pale pink. The original squamous epithelium of the vagina and ectocervix has four layers **(Figures 2-3A and B)**.

1. *The basal layer:* The basal layer is a single row of immature cells with a large nuclei and a small amount of cytoplasm. The basal cell layer is arranged on the basement membrane. The basal cells divide and differentiate into parabasal, intermediate and superficial cells. As the cells mature from basal epithelium to superficial layers, there is a gradual increase in cytoplasm and a reduction in nuclear size.
2. *The parabasal layer:* The parabasal layer includes two to four rows of immature cells that have normal mitotic figures.
3. *The intermediate layer* contains four to six rows of cells, polyhedral in shape with large amount of cytoplasm. The cells are separated by an intercellular space and the glycogen content is increased.
4. *The superficial layer* has five to eight rows of flattened cells with large amounts of cytoplasm containing glycogen. The nucleus is small, uniform and pyknotic.

These cells detach from the surface (exfoliation) and these cells form the basis for the Papanicolaou (Pap) testing.

In postmenopausal women, the cells do not mature beyond the parabasal layer; therefore, multiple layers of cells are not seen. As a result, the squamous epithelium becomes thin and atrophic. Therefore, it appears pale and brittle with sub-epithelial petechiae and it is easily prone to trauma **(Figure 2-4)**.

COLUMNAR EPITHELIUM

The endocervix of the cervix is lined by a single layer of columnar cells, which show dark staining round the nucleus at the base with mucus on the top. On naked-eye inspection, the columnar epithelium appears red, because the color of the underlying stromal vasculature is transmitted through a single layer of columnar epithelium. The columnar epithelium

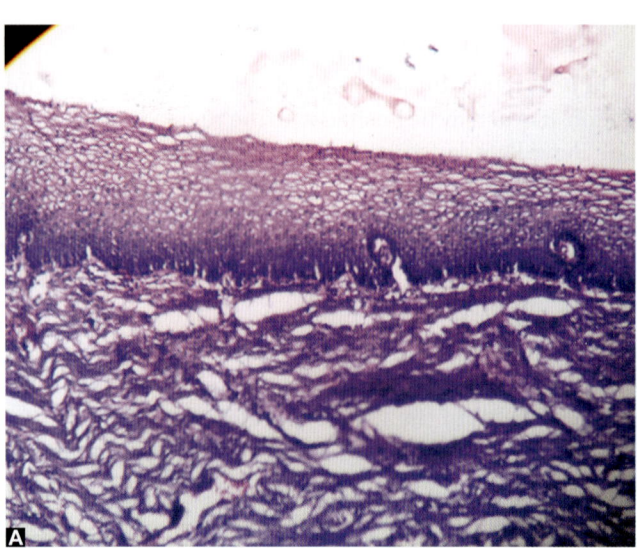

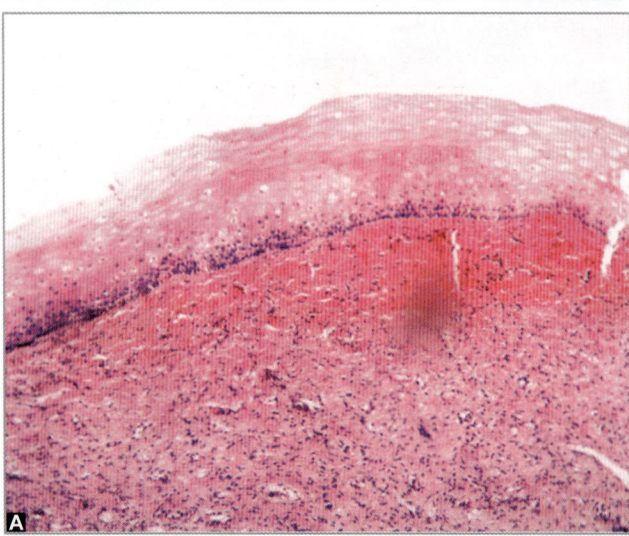

Figures 2-3A and B: Squamous epithelium of normal cervix

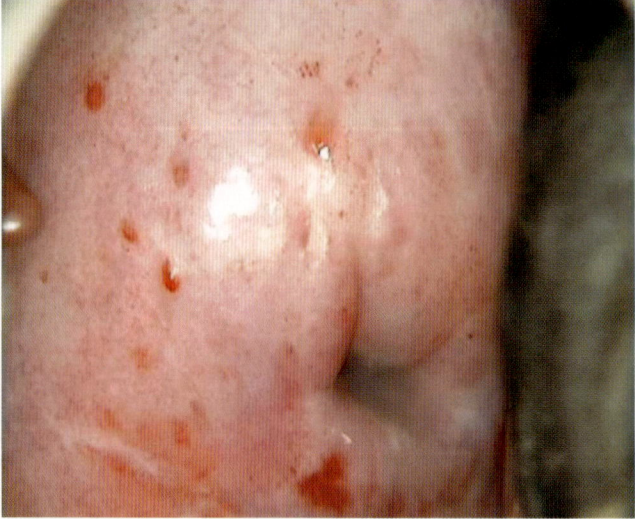

Figure 2-4: Postmenopausal cervix with petechial hemorrhages

also buries into the stroma through the basement membrane producing endocervical ridges and crypts. These infoldings, when covered by squamous metaplasia, give an appearance of gland openings **(Figure 2-5)**. The mouth of these gland openings can get occluded, the mucus collecting within the glands forming what are called nabothian cysts **(Figure 2-6)**.

Occasionally, there may be localized proliferation of endocervical glands to produce what is called endocervical polyp **(Figures 2-7A and B)**.

SHEDDING OF CELLS IN VARIOUS AGE GROUPS[7]

Depending upon the age of the individual and endocrine status, the cytological picture also varies.

Different hormones have different effects on the cellular morphology, namely the degree of maturation, relationship of one cell to another (stickiness, singleness), their cellular contents, and their overall cellular shape (crinkling, flatness).

The exfoliated cells from the cervix include parabasal cells, intermediate and superficial cells. Two morphological features separate these three cell types.

Cytoplasm

- Parabasal cells have thick cytoplasm.
- Intermediate and superficial cell types have wafer-thin cytoplasm.

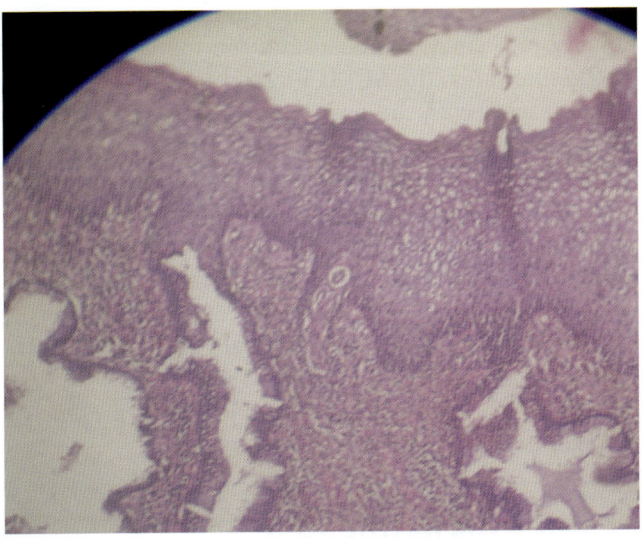

Figure 2-5: Squamous epithelium with endocervical glands

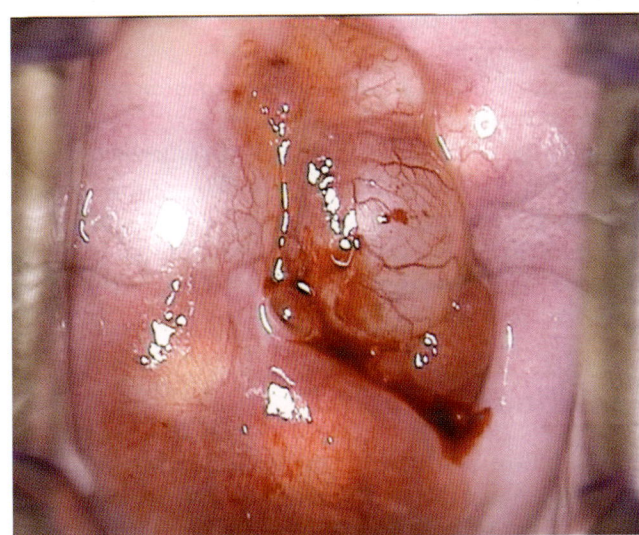

Figure 2-6: Nabothian cyst

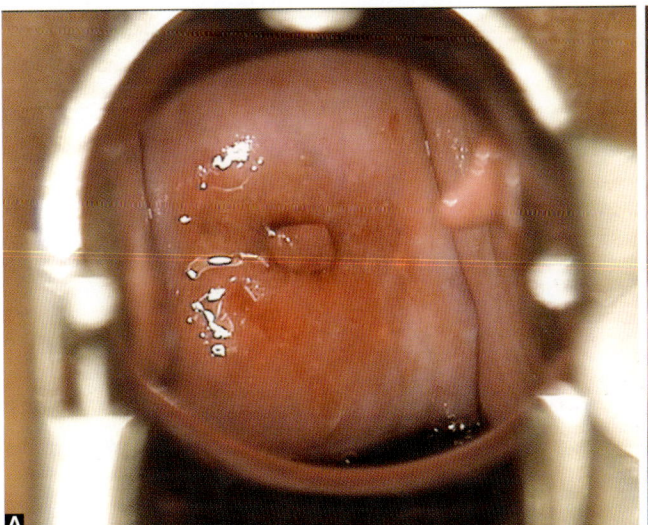
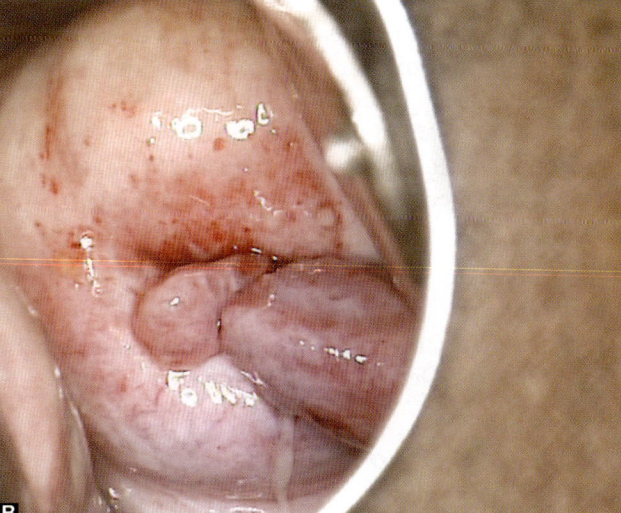

Figures 2-7A and B: Endocervical polyp

Nuclear Pattern

- In intermediate cell type, the nucleus is metabolic (plump, vesicular, intact chromatin pattern).
- In superficial cells, the nucleus is pyknotic (small, chromatin pattern is lost, hyperchromatic).

EXPOSURE TO ESTROGEN

When exposed to estrogen, the epithelium thickens and proliferates with intermediate and superficial cells. When the exposure to estrogen is more, the percentage of superficial cells is increased. Cellular degeneration and inflammation are reduced or cleared and smear appears 'clean' with cells lying flat and distributed singly.

Exposure to Progestogens

When exposed to progestogens, the epithelium proliferates and matures to intermediate cell stage.

When the epithelium is primed with sufficient estrogen and in the presence of Doderlein's bacillis, cytolysis occurs. Edges of the intermediate cell cytoplasm crinkle or curl up and the cells appear to be sticky and clumped together in masses. The background is messy with mucus, neutrophils and cellular debris.

Childhood Period

In the childhood period, the epithelium is thin and the exfoliated cells are parabasal or intermediate cells (Appearance of superficial cells is abnormal).

Reproductive Age

- In the first half of the cycle, superficial cells predominate with single layer of clear cells. This is the ideal time to take Pap smear.
- In the second half of the cycle, the intermediate cells predominate; they are crowded and curl at the borders. Taking Pap smear during this time is best avoided.

Pregnancy

During pregnancy, there is exaggerated intermediate cell picture due to high levels of progesterone in the body.

Postpartum Period

In the postpartum period, the smears appear atrophic and almost all cells are parabasal.

Postmenopausal Period

In the postmenopausal period, two patterns of cells are seen:
- Intermediate cell atrophy with predominance of intermediate cells and is usually asymptomatic.
- Parabasal cell atrophy (Teleatrophy). At this stage, the tissues get inflamed and infected from organisms, which are usually nonpathogenic. Small amounts of oestrogen will quickly mature the epithelium and heal the infection.

In the postmenopausal period, the superficial cells should be less than 10%.

THE SQUAMOCOLUMNAR JUNCTION (SCJ)

The SCJ is a dynamic point that changes in response to puberty, pregnancy, menopause and hormonal stimulation. In the neonates, the SCJ is located on the ectocervix. At menarche, with the production of estrogen, there is accumulation of glycogen in the cells. Lactobacilli present in the vagina act on the glycogen to lower the pH, which stimulates the sub-columnar reserve cells to undergo metaplasia.[8] Metaplasia advances from the original SCJ inward, towards the external OS and over the columnar villi, eventually forming an active new SCJ. The area between the original SCJ and the new physiologically active SCJ is called the transformation zone (TZ) **(Figure 2-8)**.

The transformation zone is identified by the presence of gland openings and nabothian cysts.

Metaplastic Epithelium

The metaplastic epithelium found at the SCJ begins in the subcolumnar reserve cells. The reserve cells, under the

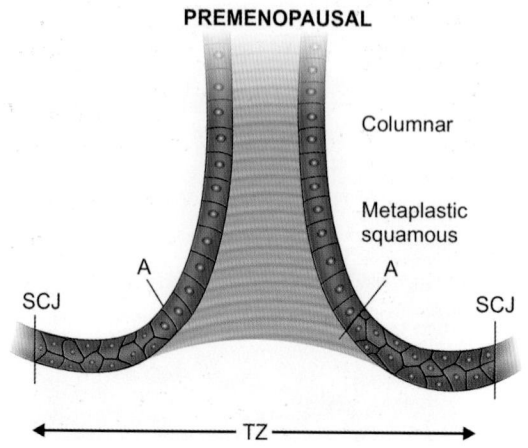

Figure 2-8: Metaplastic squamous epithelium, SCJ and TZ

stimulation of low pH of vagina, proliferate and lift the columnar epithelium.

The metaplastic process begins at the tips of columnar villi and proceeds into the cervical clefts. However, the deeper clefts may not be completely replaced by the metaplastic epithelium. As a result, mucus-secreting columnar epithelium is trapped under the squamous epithelium. This results in gland openings and nabothian cysts. The immature metaplastic cells have large nuclei with small amount of cytoplasm without glycogen. As the metaplastic cells mature normally, they produce glycogen, eventually forming the four layers of squamous epithelium. Once the metaplastic epithelium matures and forms glycogen, it is called the healed TZ and is relatively resistant to oncogenic stimulation.

BLOOD SUPPLY TO THE CERVIX

The arterial supply to the cervix is from the descending cervical branch of uterine artery. These vessels divide and subdivide as they near the external os of the cervix. Therefore, in procedures like cervical biopsy, the bleeding is minimal and can be controlled by packing. In large loop excision of the transformation zone (LLETZ), the depth of cone may be as long as 1.5–2 cm. In these procedures, the active bleeding can be safely coagulated. In cold knife cone biopsy, the descending cervical branch is ligated on either side to minimize blood loss.

NERVE SUPPLY

The nerve supply to the cervix is derived from the hypogastric plexus. There are very few sensory fibers in the ectocervix and is plenty in the endocervix. Therefore, any procedure on the ectocervix such as biopsy, cryotherapy are well tolerated without local anesthesia. Procedures like LLETZ would need paracervical block. The endocervix has an abundance of sympathetic and parasympathetic fibers. Therefore, any manipulation of cervix, such as uterine sounding or endocervical curettage can cause severe pain by stimulating these nerve endings.

Gland openings and nabothian cysts mark the original SCJ and the outer edge of the original SCJ
- Metaplasia is most active during menarche and pregnancy
- In most cases CIN originates as a single focus in the TZ at the advancing SCJ
- Once CIN occurs, it progresses laterally to involve the entire TZ, but usually does not replace the original squamous epithelium
- Proximally, CIN involves the cervical clefts and tends to have most severe CIN lesions, therefore, should be destroyed completely
- The entire SCJ with early metaplastic cells is susceptible to oncogenic stimuli

Chapter 3

Etiology and Risk Factors for Cervical Carcinoma

The occurrence of cervical cancer depends upon three important factors **(Figure 3-1)**:
- Active metaplasia in the transformation zone (TZ)
- Exposure to oncogen
- Immune status of the individual.

METAPLASIA IN THE TRANSFORMATION ZONE

Cervical intraepithelial neoplasia (CIN) arises in an area of metaplasia in the TZ. During menarche and pregnancy, the metaplasia is very active. In adolescent girls and in pregnancy high levels of estrogen exposes the columnar epithelium of the endocervix onto the ectocervix. This results in exposure of the columnar epithelium to the vaginal acidity. This induces metaplastic changes in the cervix, during which time, it is vulnerable to oncogens. Long-term use of oral contraceptive pills also results in exposing the columnar epithelium onto the ectocervix. In multiparous women, due to cervical injury, ectropion and chronic cervicitis the columnar epithelium is exposed to the vaginal acidity.

Therefore, initiating sexual activity before the age of 16, young age at first pregnancy, use of OC pills and high parity are important risk factors for the development of carcinoma of cervix. First intercourse before 16 years of age is associated with a twofold increased risk of cervical cancer compared with that for women whose first intercourse occurred after the age of 20 years.[9] Studies have shown that long-term oral contraceptive users (>5 years) have about a twofold increased risk of cervical carcinoma compared with that of non-users. Use of barrier methods has been shown to lower the risk of cervical carcinoma, by reducing the exposure to infectious agents. There is a linear dose-response relationship between contraceptive use and cervical cancer, but the relationship tends to disappear with time after OC pill cessation.[10]

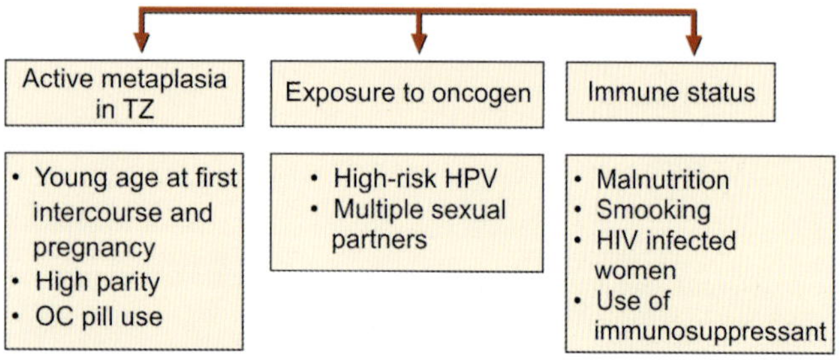

> After menopause, a woman undergoes little metaplasia and is at a lower risk of developing CIN.
> CIN is most likely to begin either soon after menarche or after pregnancy, when metaplasia is most active.

EXPOSURE TO ONCOGENS

Cervical carcinoma is a disease related to sexual activity. The primary underlying cause of cervical carcinoma is human papillomavirus (HPV), which is the most common sexually transmitted disease. HPV infection affects 75–80% of sexually active women at least once in their lifetime. Women generally contract HPV infection at the onset of sexual activity in their teens, 20s or 30s. But, majority of infections

Active metaplasia in TZ	Exposure to oncogen	Immune status
• Young age at first intercourse and pregnancy • High parity • OC pill use	• High-risk HPV • Multiple sexual partners	• Malnutrition • Smooking • HIV infected women • Use of immunosuppressant

Figure 3-1: Eetiology and risk factors for cervical carcinoma

Etiology and Risk Factors for Cervical Carcinoma

are transient, and by some mechanism, the infection spontaneously clears from the body. However, 5% of women eventually develop cervical carcinoma due to persistence of infection with high risk type of HPV. The woman's chances of contracting HPV infection are more when she or her partner has multiple sexual partners. Cancer cervix is also high when the husbands had previous partners with cancer cervix or when the husbands suffered from cancer of the penis. There are two types of HPV infection. The low risk type 6, 11 and 42 are usually associated with mild dysplasia and condyloma. Nearly 15 (oncogenic) high risk types have been identified **(Figure 3-2)** and they belong to two important phytogenetically related families and are associated with severe dysplasia and invasive carcinoma. Those related to HPV-16, (Types-31-33,-35,-52 and -58) and those related to HPV-18, (Types-39,-45,-59 and -68) **(Figure 3-3)** HPV-16 and -18 cause 70% of cervical cancers and HPV-45 and -31 are responsible for another 10% of the cases.

IMMUNE STATUS OF THE INDIVIDUAL

The development of the cervical cancer is also influenced by the immune status of the individual. The immune response is poor in women from poor socioeconomic group due to malnutrition, deficiency of vitamin E, vitamin C and micronutrients. Women suffering from HIV infection, who are on renal transplant with immune suppressor drugs are also highly susceptible. The Centres for Disease Control and Prevention have described cervical cancer as an acquired immunodeficiency syndrome (AIDS) in patients infected with HIV. In these cases, cell-mediated immunity appears to be a factor in the development of cervical cancer.[11] Immunocompromised women may not only be at high risk for the disease, but also demonstrate rapid progression from preinvasive to invasive lesion. Reproductive tract hygiene, smoking, infections and lower socioeconomic status are other risk factors for cervical cancer.

SMOKING AND CERVICAL CARCINOMA

Studies have shown that the risk of developing cervical cancer is highest in long term and high intensity smokers and "ever smoking" was associated with a significant two-fold increase in the risk of cervical carcinoma. Tobacco metabolites—nicotine and continine are present in high levels in the cervical mucus of smokers. These have genotoxic and immunosuppressive effects. Moreover, smokers show reduced intake of dietary antioxidants.[12]

Co-infection with Sexually Transmitted Infectious Agents and Cervical Carcinoma.

Studies have shown that cervical inflammation may be associated with high-grade lesions and may be a co-factor for high grade cervical lesions in women infected with oncogenic HPV.[13] Inflammation is a relatively non-specific physiological response to tissue injury caused by exogenous factors such as microbial infections and chemical irritants. Inflammation in response to chronic infection triggers migration of natural killer cells and phagocytes (neutrophils and macrophages) to the infected site. These cells release inflammatory mediators (IL-1 and IL-8). There is also production of nonspecific protective antimicrobial oxidants that can also cause oxidative damage to host DNA leading to cancer.[14] IARC multicentric study found a 2-fold increase in risk of cervical cancer in the presence of antibodies to C – Trachomatis or to HSV-2 infections.

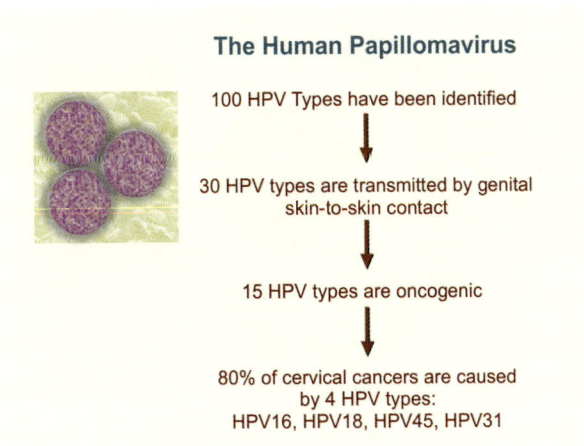

Figure 3-2: Human papilloma virus

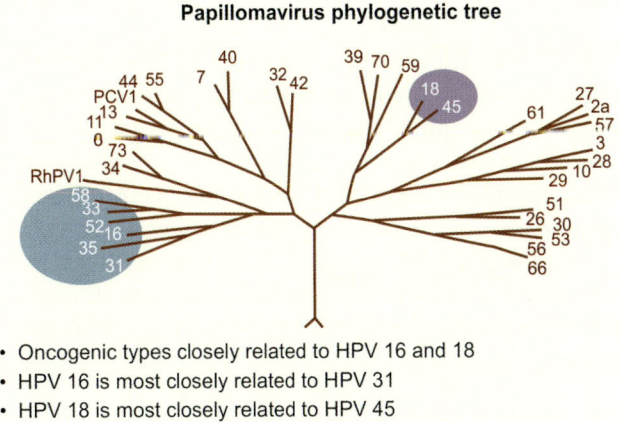

Figure 3-3: Papillomavirus phylogenetic tree

Chapter 4

Human Papillomavirus and Cervical Carcinoma

ONCOGENESIS OF HPV

Human papillomaviruses (HPVs) are small DNA viruses that infect various epithelial tissues and mucosal membranes. More than 100 types of HPVs have been described. They share a circular DNA genome of 8000 base pairs organized into an early, late and long control regions. The early region encodes for proteins E1, E2, E3, E4, E5, E6 and E7, which influence viral infection and replication. Two genes from the early control regions E6 and E7 are essential for HPV-induced process of cellular transformation, and two genes from the late control regions L1 and L2 encode the viral capsid protein. When the HPV DNA integrates into the host genome, there is breakage at E1 and E2 regions and this loss of E2 causes uncontrolled expression of E6 and E7 oncoproteins. When there is continuous expression of E6 and E7 oncoproteins by high-risk HPVs, there are genomic aberrations in the host cells, which can lead to malignant conversion. The virus particles promote the proliferation of infected cells by disrupting the stability of cell DNA and causing chromosomal instability. The expressed oncoproteins E6 and E7 respectively bind and inactivate cell tumor suppression proteins p53 and pRB (retinoblastoma tumor suppressor genes), and are essential for malignant transformation. Inhibition of p53 prevents cell cycle arrest and cellular apoptosis, which normally occurs when damaged DNA is present. Inhibition of RB results in unregulated cellular proliferation. In most cases, innate and adaptive immune responses control HPV infection. However, the high-risk type viruses have the ability to escape immune defenses by interfering with the interferon pathway, resulting in persistent infection and progression to neoplasia.

According to the ability of the virus to promote malignant transformation, HPV is classified into low- and high-risk types.

HIGH-RISK AND LOW-RISK-TYPE HPVs (FIGURES 4-1 AND 4-2)

The low-risk-type 6, 11 and 42 are usually associated with mild dysplasia and condyloma. Nearly 15 (oncogenic) high-risk types have been identified and they belong to two important phytogenetically related families and are associated with severe dysplasia and invasive carcinoma. These oncogenic HPV types are members of either A7 (HPV 18, 39, 45, 59, 68, 70 and 85) or A9 (HPV 16, 31, 33, 35, 52, 58 and 68).

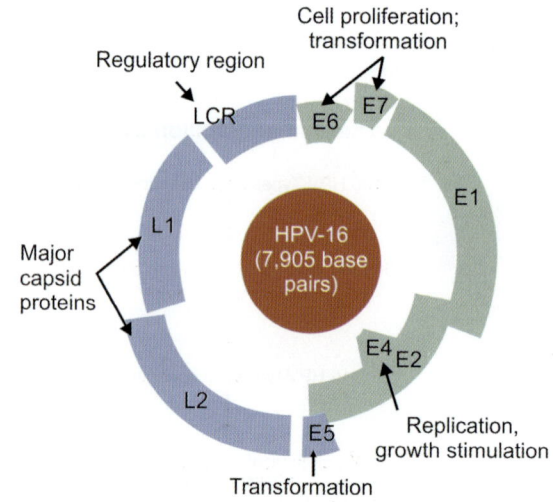

Figure 4-1: Normal cell cycle

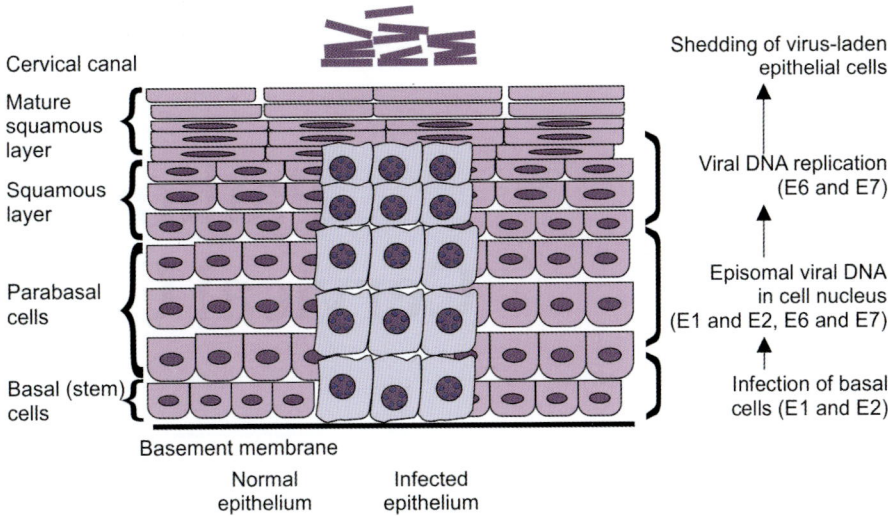

Figure 4-2: Lifecycle of HPV in the cervix

High-risk HPV-16 and HPV-18 are associated with more than 99% of cervical carcinomas. HPV-16 accounts for 50–60% of all cervical cancer cases, followed by HPV-18 (10–20%). HPV-45 (4–8%) and HPV-31 (1–5%).[15]

The oncogenic risk of the HPV types appears to be related to the binding affinity of their E6 and E7 proteins to p53 and Rb respectively. E6 and E7 proteins from high-risk HPV bind with high affinity to p53 and Rb respectively, whereas low-risk HPV E6 and E7 proteins bind with very low affinity.

The HPV Cell Cycle[16] (Figure 4-2)

- The HPV lifecycle is restricted to the cervical epithelium; there is no viremia.
- The virus is thought to infect the basal cell layer of the epithelium via microabrasions.
- It then uses the host cell machinery to replicate viral DNA and express virally encoded proteins.
- The HPV genome encodes eight genes:
  - Six encode the 'early' or nonstructural proteins (E1, E2, E4, E5, E6 and E7)
  - Two encode the 'late' or structural proteins (L1 and L2).
- Finally, new virus particles are assembled in the upper layers of the epithelium and virus is released with the cells as they are shed from the epithelial surface.

Chapter 5
Pathogenesis of Cervical Carcinoma

HPV infection plays an essential role in the pathogenesis of cervical carcinoma. Most women are exposed to and infected with HPV shortly after sexual activity.

- The immature basal cells of the squamous epithelium are the target cells for an initial HPV infection. The HPV virus reaches these cells through microabrasion in the epithelium **(Figure 5-1)**.
- The viral replication is tightly linked to the differentiating state of the virally infected epithelial cells. As the immature basal cells differentiate and mature into superficial squamous cells, along with the host genome, the viral DNA replication also takes place.
- The copies of DNA genome is low in the basal cell nuclei and virally encoded proteins are expressed at very low levels. As a result, HPV infected basal cells show no specific cytologic histological changes and cannot be distinguished from the uninfected cells. This stage of the disease is referred to as latent infection.
- As HPV-infected epithelial cells differentiate and move upwards in the epithelium, viral transcription dramatically increases.
- When infection occurs, replication of viral particles requires mature squamous keratinocytes.
- Infectious virus is eventually released as the differentiated cells are shed from the epithelium.

In most women, after a period of time, immunity develops against HPV, and productive viral infection ceases. These women eventually become HPV DNA negative. In some HPV-infected women, viral gene expression is not linked to the differentiation of infected epithelial cells.

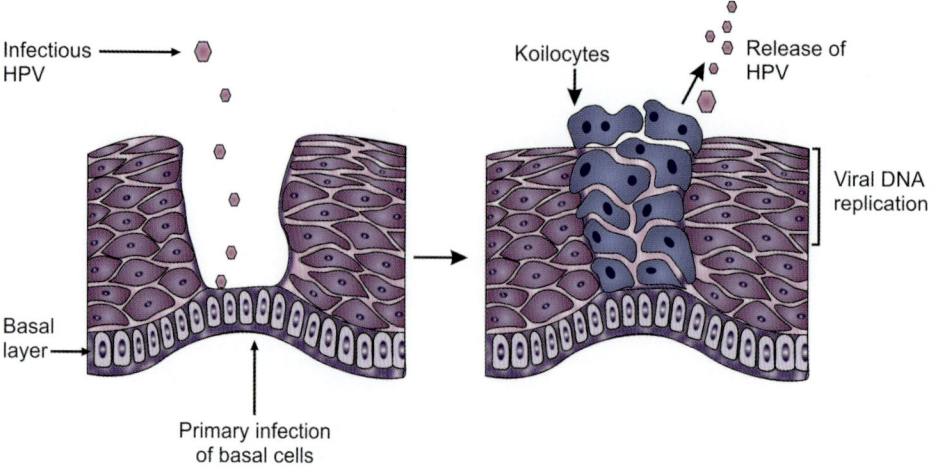

Figure 5-1: Phases of HPV infection

Instead, there is dramatic expression of E6 and E7 HPV in the lower layer of the epithelium, which results in the disruption of normal cell cycle regulation and there is genetic instability. This genetic instability results in aberrant mitotic events, changes in number and structure of chromosomes, further producing changes in overall DNA content, referred to as aneuploidy. And this genetic instability plays a critical role in the development of cervical cancer.[17]

Cervical carcinoma is a disease related to sexual activity. Women generally contract HPV in their teens, 20s or 30s. But, by some mechanism, the infection spontaneously clears from the body. Most HPV infection in young women is transient. Only in a small proportion of women, the infection is persistent with high-risk types of HPV. Peak levels of high-risk types of HPV occur in 20–25% of women between 20 and 24 years of age. However, for those over the age of 25 years, persistent high-risk types are found only in 4–5% of cases.[18] Persistent infection with HPV 16 and 18 is associated with highly increased risk for subsequent development of invasive cervical carcinoma.[19] Factors which lead to HPV persistence are: HPV type (greatest risk is seen with HPV-16), increasing age, smoking, immunosuppression, inflammation and genetic factors.

Chapter 6

Progression and Regression of CIN Lesions

There is often a long interval between exposure to HPV and the development of cervical cancer which may take up to 30 years. About 90% of low-grade lesions regress spontaneously and without intervention. However, almost 50% of cases with high-grade lesions progress to cervical cancer **(Figure 6-1)**.

Ostor, in 1993 reviewed studies on natural history of CIN lesions. The investigator concluded that spontaneous regression occurred in 57%, 43% and 32% of cases for CIN1, CIN2, and CIN3 lesions respectively. 1% of CIN lesions, 5% of CIN2 lesions, and >12% of CIN3 lesions progressed to invasive cervical cancer during follow-up[21] **(Table 6-1)**.

Table 6-1: Summary of the natural history of CIN lesions

	Regression	Progression	Progression to CIS	Progression to invasive carcinoma
CIN1	57%	32%	11%	1%
CIN2	43%	35%	22%	5%
CIN3	32%	56%		12%

It is also now recognized that high-grade CIN lesions (CIN2, 3) also develop quickly after an incident infection with high grades of types of HPV and not necessarily preceded by CIN1 lesions.[22]

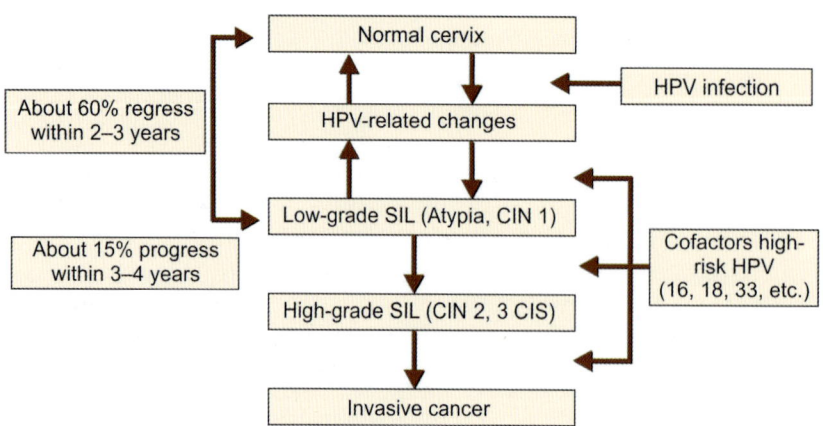

Figure 6-1: Natural History of Cervical Cancer (Adapted from reference 20)

Chapter 7

Histology of Cervical Intraepithelial Neoplasia

The abnormal cervical epithelium shows varying degrees of immaturity and nuclear abnormalities. The proportion of the thickness of epithelium showing immaturity and undifferentiated cells is used for grading of CIN. In more severe degrees of CIN, greater proportion of the thickness of epithelium shows undifferentiated cells with only a small narrow layer of mature differentiated cells on the surface. Nuclear abnormalities such as enlarged nucleus, increased nuclear cytoplasmic ratio, increased intensity of nuclear staining (hyperchromasia) and variation in nuclear size are also assessed when the diagnosis is made.

There is a strong correlation between epithelium revealing immaturity and the degree of nuclear abnormality. As the severity of CIN increases, the epithelium becomes less differentiated, the number of mitotic figures increases and are seen in the superficial layers of the epithelium. (Mitotic figures are seen in the dividing cells; they are infrequent in normal epithelium and, if present, are seen in the parabasal layers.)

CIN1 LESIONS (FIGURES 7-1A TO C)

In CIN1, there is good maturation, with minimal nuclear abnormalities and few mitotic figures. There is loss of normal progressive cellular differentiation in the lower third of the epithelium and the normal cell maturation is maintained in the upper 2/3rds of the epithelial layer. Undifferentiated cells are confined to the deeper layers (lower third) of the epithelium. Epithelial changes due to HPV infection may be observed in the full thickness of the epithelium.

CIN2 LESIONS (FIGURES 7-2A TO C)

CIN2 lesions are characterized by dysplastic cellular changes restricted to the lower two-thirds of the epithelium. Mitotic figures may be seen throughout the involved thickness of the epithelium.

In some areas, a small strip in the lower 1/3rd is involved; other areas showing involvement of nearly 50% of the epithelium (Figure 7-3).

CIN3 LESIONS (FIGURES 7-4A TO C)

In CIN3, differentiation and stratification may be totally absent or present only in the superficial quarter of the epithelium with numerous mitotic figures. Nuclear abnormalities and loss of polarity are seen through the entire thickness of the epithelium.

Arrow is indicating involvement of more than 2/3rd of cell thickness with dysplastic cells. Apoptotic cells are also seen (Figure 7-5).

In high-grade lesions, the lesions are more immature. Normally, the basal layer of the squamous epithelium is two-cell layer thick. In high-grade CIN lesions, there is marked proliferation of basal cells with increased nuclear cytoplasmic ratio and variability in nuclear size showing marked atypia. The cells show marked mitotic activity and basaloid cells replace the normal cells in the superficial layer. (In low-grade lesions, only the basal layer is dedifferentiated and the upper layers retain their cytoplasmic differentiation.) Figure 7-6.

16 A Practical Approach to Cervical Cancer Screening Techniques

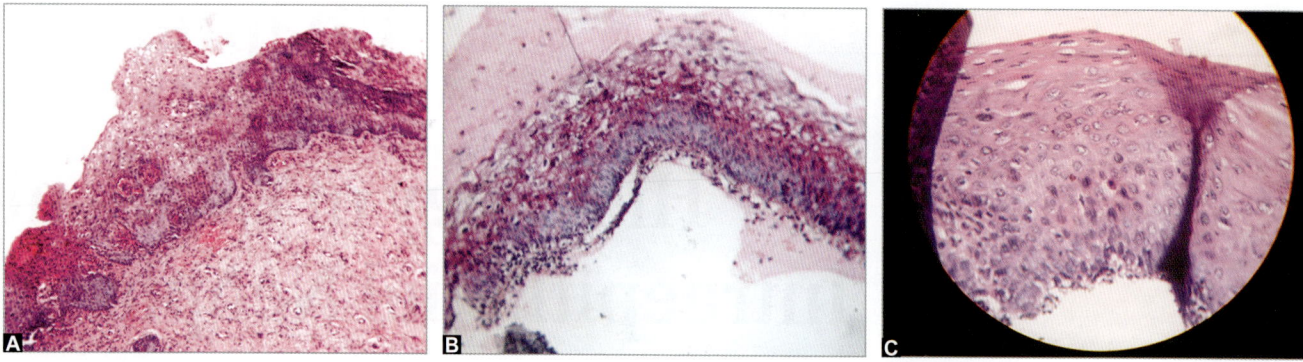

Figures 7-1A to C: CIN1 lesions; H and E—low power; H and E—high power. There is an involvement of lower 1/3rd with minimal nuclear abnormalities. The upper 2/3rd shows good maturation of cells

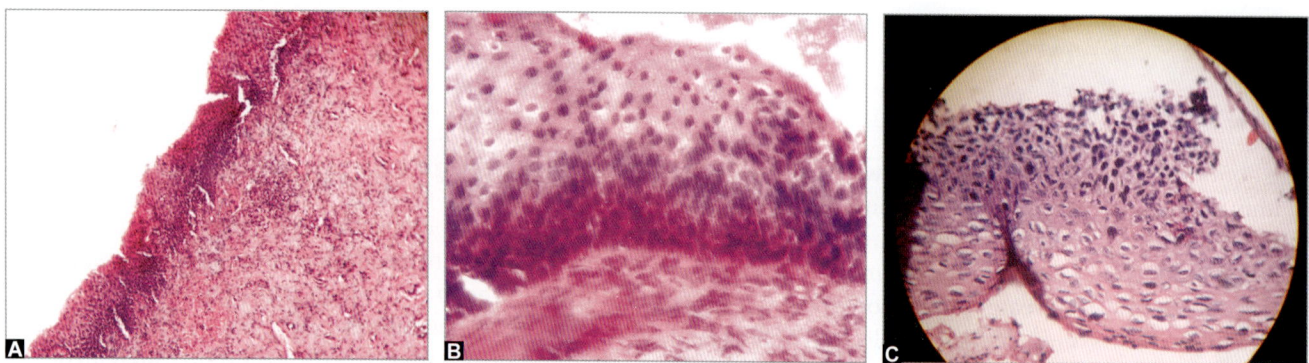

Figures 7-2A to C: HPE of CIN2 lesions: HPE—low power; HPE—high power. Dysplastic cellular changes are seen in the lower 2/3rd of the epithelium. Polarity is lost and nuclear enlargement and hyperchromasia are seen in the affected epithelium

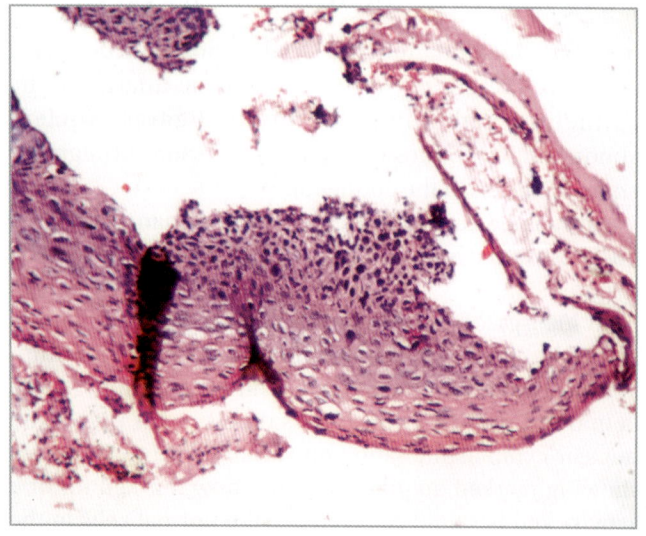

Figure 7-3: HPE of CIN1, 2 lesions – High power

Adenocarcinoma In Situ (AIS) (Figure 7-7)

In AIS, normal columnar epithelium is replaced by abnormal epithelium showing loss of polarity, increased cell size, nuclear hyperchromasia, mitotic activity, reduction of cytoplasmic mucin expression and cellular stratification and piling.

Abnormal branching and budding with intraluminal papillary projections lacking stromal core may also be observed. The majority of AIS are seen in the TZ. And AIS may be associated with CIN of the squamous epithelium in nearly 2/3rds of cases.

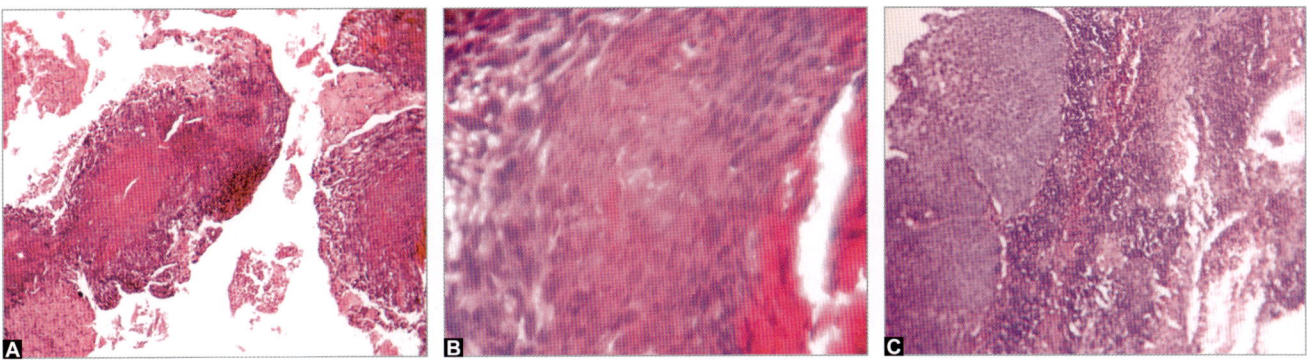

Figures 7-4A to C: CIN3 lesions

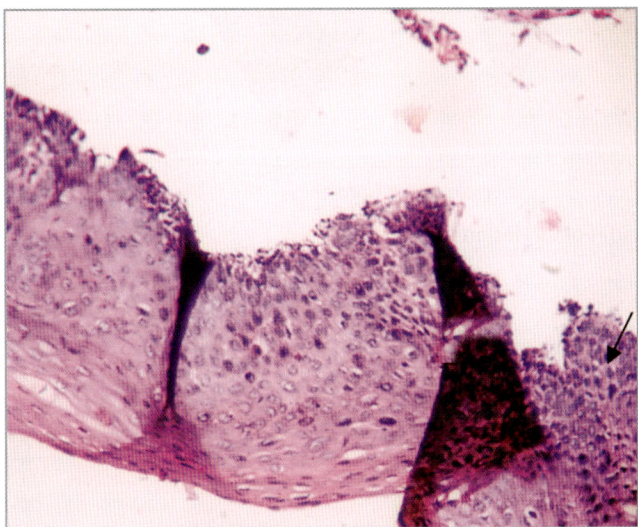

Figure 7-5: CIN2, 3 changes

Histopathology of Invasive Cancers

According to the international histological classification, the malignant tumors of the cervix are classified into epithelial and nonepithelial tumors.

A. Epithelial Tumors

1. *Squamous cell carcinomas (Epidermoid carcinomas)*
   These carcinomas constitute 80–95% of all tumors.
   Here nests of neoplastic squamous cells invade into the subepithelial stroma. The neoplastic cells are of different shape, they are in groups, and the nuclei are large and irregular with hyperchromasia. In well-differentiated squamous carcinoma of the cervix, the most prominent feature is the presence of keratin pearls. Keratin pearls are eosiniphilic, surrounded by epithelial cells. Based on the degree of differentiation, morphologically, the squamous cell carcinomas are divided into:
   - Large cell keratinizing type (well-differentiated) **(Figure 7-8)**
   - Large cell nonkeratinizing (moderately differentiated) **(Figure 7-9)**
   - Small cell nonkeratinizing (poorly differentiated) **(Figure 7-10)**.

   Prognosis is better with large cell keratinizing tumors. Small cell tumors are anaplastic and they behave aggressively with poor prognosis.
   Another variant of squamous cell carcinoma is verrucous carcinoma, which is locally invasive and the tumor metastasis is rare. The tumor is exophytic and is often mistaken for large cervical condylomas.

2. *Adenocarcinomas (Figure 7-11)*
   Adenocarcinomas arise from the endocervical glands or from the remnants of wolffian ducts. These may be of:
   - Endocervical type
   - Endometrial type
   - Clear cell adenocarcinomas
3. Adenosquamous carcinomas
4. Undifferentiated cancer.

B. Nonepithelial Tumors

- Sarcomas—leiomyosarcoma
  - Embryonal rhabdomyosarcoma (sarcoma botyroids in children)
  Mixed Müllerian tumor
- Melanomas—these are rare tumors and they simulate melanomas elsewhere. Prognosis depends on the depth of invasion.
- Neuroendocrine tumors—carcinoid tumors can also occur

18 A Practical Approach to Cervical Cancer Screening Techniques

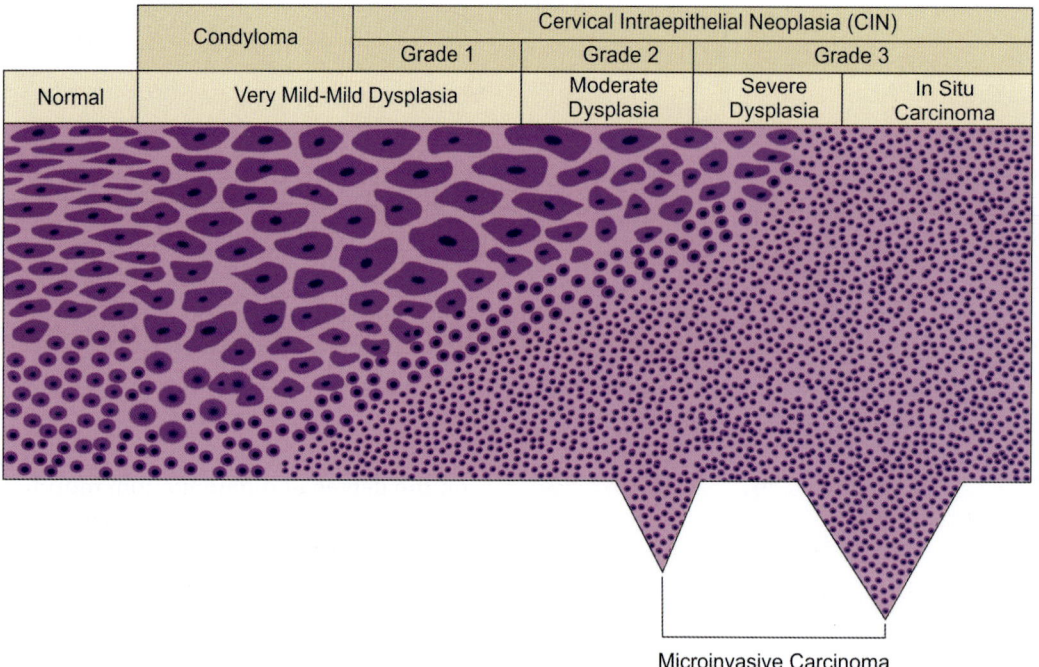

Figure 7-6: Different grades of CIN lesions

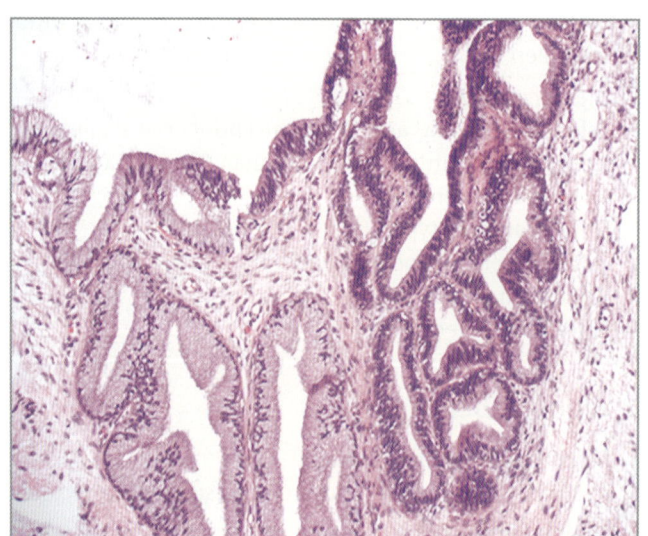

Figure 7-7: Adenocarcinoma in situ

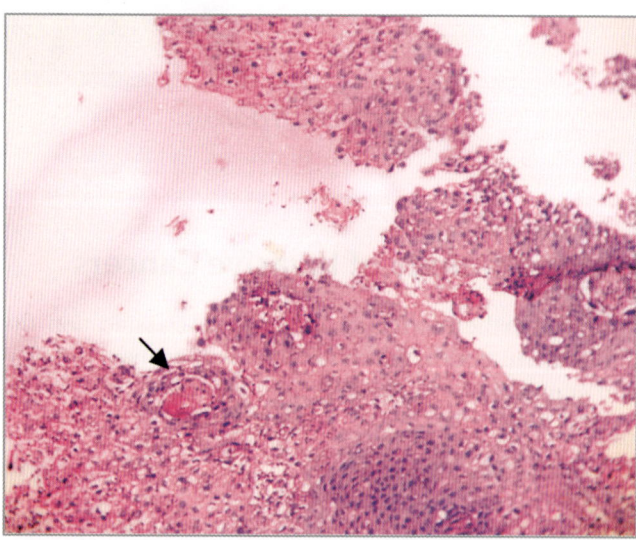

Figure 7-8: Well-differentiated squamous cell carcinoma of the cervix. Keratin pearl is indicated by an arrow

Histology of Cervical Intraepithelial Neoplasia

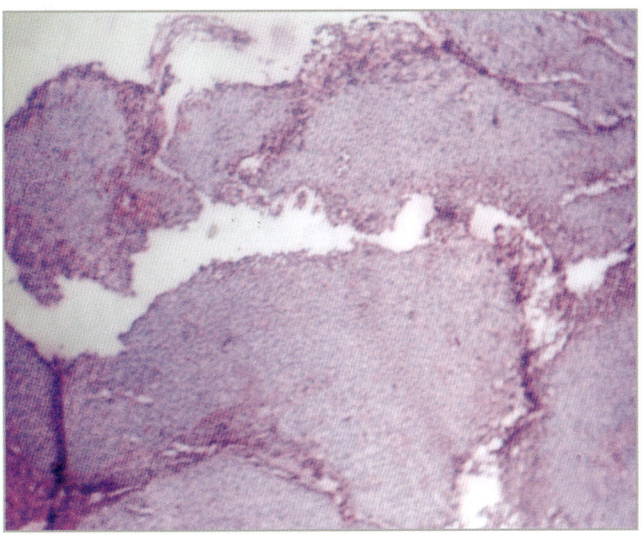

Figure 7-9: Moderately differentiated squamous cell carcinoma of the cervix

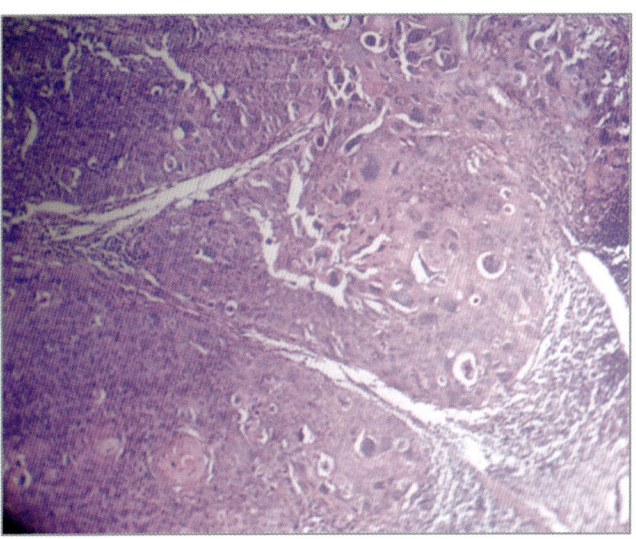

Figure 7-10: Poorly differentiated carcinoma of the cervix

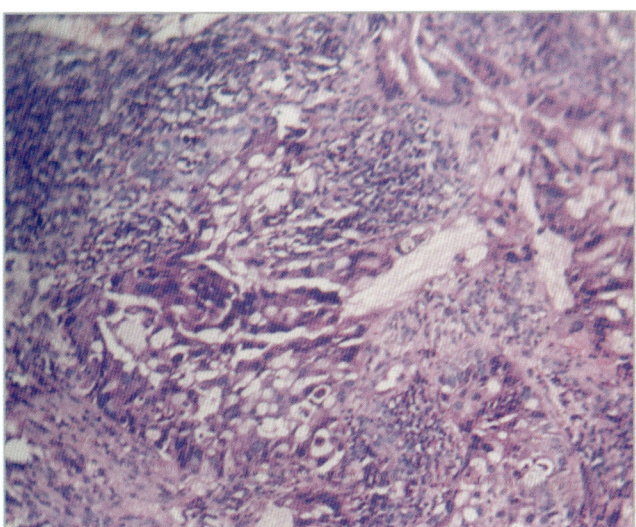

Figure 7-11: Adenocarcinoma of the cervix

Chapter 8

Screening Tests for Cervical Carcinoma

CRITERIA FOR A SCREENING TEST

An ideal screening test is the one that is:
- Minimally invasive
- Easy to perform
- Acceptable to the subject
- Cost effective
- Effective in diagnosing the disease process in its pre-invasive or early invasive stage, when the disease process is more easily treatable and curable.

In all probability, cervical cancer is the only gynecological cancer that satisfies the well-recognized WHO criteria for implementation of a screening program.
- The natural history of the disease is known and there is existence of well-defined premalignant lesions
- There is a long latent period during which premalignant change or occult cancer can be detected and effectively treated, thereby altering the natural history of the disease
- There is a clearly defined viral etiology, which could be incorporated as a marker in mass screening programs
- There is an easy and direct access of the uterine cervix for examination and sampling
- Effective treatments are available for the premalignant change

SCREENING TECHNIQUES FOR CERVICAL CANCER INCLUDE THE FOLLOWING:

- Conventional exfoliative cervicovaginal cytology, i.e. the cervical (Pap) smear
- Fluid sampling techniques with automated thin layer preparation (liquid-based cytology)
- Automated cervical screening techniques
- HPV testing
- Visual inspection of cervix after applying Lugol's iodine (VILI) or acetic acid (VIA)
- Polar probe
- Laser-induced fluorescence
- Speculoscopy
- Cervicography.

CERVICAL CYTOLOGY

The Papanicolaou Smear

The Pap test is a simple cytological technique to detect pre-invasive stage of cervical carcinoma. It was in 1928, George N Papanicolaou, an Anatomist introduced cytology in the diagnosis of cervical carcinoma, which came into clinical practice in 1940. Subsequently, J Ernest Ayre, a Gynecologist introduced wooden spatula, the Ayre's spatula to collect cells from the transformation zone.

The reporting of cervical smear has gone through various systems from 1954 through 2001 **(Table 8-1)**.
- The first system of reporting of cervical cytology was devised by George N Papanicolaou in 1954 and the classification was based on the degree of certainty that malignant cells were present.
- Subsequently in 1968, based on the morphologic criteria, WHO introduced a descriptive terminology with various grades of dysplasia, namely mild, moderate, severe dysplasia and invasive carcinoma.
- It was in 1978 that Richart coined the name cervical intra-epithelial neoplasia (CIN). The CIN terminology divided the precursor lesion into three groups, namely

Table 8-1: Reporting of cervical cytology

Papanicolaou Class System (1954)	Descriptive (1968)	CIN (1978)	Bethesda System (1988)
Class 1	Negative for malignant cells	Negative	Within normal limits
Class 2	Inflammatory atypia Squamous atypia		Reactive and reparative changes Atypical squamous cells of undetermined significance (ASCUS)
	Koilocytotic atypia		Low-grade SIL; includes condyloma
Class 3	Mild dysplasia	CIN1	Low-grade SIL; includes condyloma
	Moderate dysplasia	CIN2	High-grade SIL
	Severe dysplasia	CIN3	High-grade SIL
Class 4	Carcinoma in situ	CIN3	High-grade SIL
Class 5	Invasive carcinoma	Invasive carcinoma	Invasive carcinoma

CIN1, CIN2 and CIN3. The groups were considered to represent different stages of a single biological process, which could progress to carcinoma in situ and, therefore, cervical carcinoma. The terminology was used both in histopathology and cytopathology.

- The Bethesda system (TBS).

In cervical carcinogenesis, HPV infection is accepted as an essential early event, and these HPV-associated cervical lesions are considered as two distinct biological entities. Now it is well recognised that high-grade lesions (CIN2, 3) often develop quickly following an infection with high-risk HPV types and not necessarily preceded by CIN 1 changes. Therefore, high-grade lesions are potentially cervical cancer precursors. Whereas, not all low-grade lesions (CIN1) are neoplastic, most are self-limiting and regress spontaneously.

Therefore, based on the above biological characteristics of the lesions, in 1988, the Bethesda system of reporting was introduced. The Bethesda system replaced three levels of CIN with two levels, namely low-grade and high-grade intraepithelial lesions and this could be used to describe any squamous abnormality of the lower genital tract. As there is high spontaneous regression rate of some dysplastic lesions and the lack of predictable progression of these lesions to invasive carcinoma, the term 'squamous intraepithelial lesion' is used rather than 'Neoplasia'. In 1991, further changes were made in the Bethesda system of reporting. In 2001, during the annual meeting of the American Society for Colposcopy and Cervical Pathology (ASCCP), important changes were made and new guidelines were introduced. Currently, the 2001 (revised) Bethesda system is being used.[23]

The 2001 (Revised) Bethesda System of Reporting

The Bethesda system of reporting includes the following features:
- Whether the Pap smear is an adequate sample or not.
- Whether there are incidental changes, such as evidence of infection or reparative changes.
- Whether there is an evidence of lesion, such as low-grade, high-grade lesion, carcinoma—squamous/glandular.

The reporting is done under four major subdivisions:

I. Specimen type
   - Specify conventional Pap smear or liquid-based cytology.
II. Specimen adequacy
   - Whether satisfactory for evaluation, presence or absence of endocervical, transformation zone cells.
   - Unsatisfactory for evaluation (specify the reason).
   - Specify rejected/not processed (specify reason).
III. General categorization
   - Negative for intraepithelial lesion or malignancy
   - Epithelial cell abnormality (specify squamous or glandular).
IV. Interpretation/result.

A. Negative for Intraepithelial Lesion or Malignancy (NIL)

(Indicates no cellular evidence of neoplasia, state whether or not there are organisms or other non-neoplastic findings).
- No cellular evidence of neoplasia.
- State if evidence of infection with *Actinomyces, Trichomonas vaginalis, Candida*, suggestion of bacterial vaginosis, cellular changes with Herpes simplex virus.
- State if evidence of non-neoplastic findings, such as reactive cellular changes associated with inflammation, repair, radiation, IUCD use, atrophy and benign appearing glandular cells posthysterectomy.

B. Epithelial Cell Abnormalities

Squamous Cells

- Atypical squamous cells of undetermined significance (ASC-US).
- Atypical squamous cells—cannot exclude HSIL—(ASC-H)
- Low-grade squamous intraepithelial lesion (LSIL) (includes HPV/mild dysplasia/CIN I).
- High-grade squamous intraepithelial lesion (HSIL) (includes moderate and severe dysplasia—CIS/CIN 2 and CIN 3).
- Squamous cell carcinoma.

Glandular Cells

- Negative for glandular lesion.
- Atypical glandular cells/endocervical cells/endometrial cells (AGC-US)
- Atypical glandular/endocervical cells favoring neoplasia (AGC-H)
- Endocervical adenocarcinoma in situ
- Adenocarcinoma
    - Endocervical
    - Endometrial.

Adequacy of the Specimen

According to the TBS, before proceeding onto interpretation of the smear, the cytopathologist should check the adequacy of the smear. A smear is satisfactory for evaluation if it meets the following criteria:

- The patient and the specimens are clearly identified (slide is not broken, patient identification is adequate)
- Clinical history is available
- The sample is technically interpretable, i.e. there is adequate cellular component and not more than 50% of the cells are obscured by inflammation, debris or blood
- There is an evidence that transformation zone has been sampled shown by the presence of two clusters of endocervical cells/metaplastic cells. If the specimen shows high-grade lesions or cancer, presence or absence of endocervical cells is not reported.

> In postmenopausal women, the transformation zone is likely to be covered with mature squamous cells and the endocervical brush should be used to sample the transformation zone

> In cases of unsatisfactory smears due to infection or atrophy, treat the specific cause (antibiotics/estrogen cream) and repeat the smear in 8–12 weeks

> If the unsatisfactory smear persists, or the cervix looks suspicious, refer for colposcopy directly

SAMPLE COLLECTION FOR CERVICAL CYTOLOGY

Timing

A few points to be remembered while taking a Pap smear:

- The cytological sample should not be collected during the menstrual period
- The women should not have had intercourse or inserted anything into the vagina atleast 24 hours prior to Pap smear
- They should avoid intravaginal medication, contraceptive or douch for one week before taking Pap smear
- If there is obvious cervicitis or purulent discharge, treat the infection and collect the samples 4-6 weeks later
- Postpartum Pap smears should not be taken for atleast 8 weeks after delivery. If performed earlier, unsatisfactory smears will be reported more frequently due to inflammation and reparative changes
- In postmenopausal women, smears may be reported as atrophy, inflammation or lack of endocervical cells. In these cases, advice estrogen cream vaginally for 2–3 weeks to facilitate cell maturation. Give a medication-free interval for 7–10 days, and then repeat the smear.

Required Supplies for Sampling (Fig 8-1)

1. Cusco's speculum of varying depth and width should be available to expose the cervix adequately
2. Glass slides
3. Glass pencil
4. Fixative
5. Spatulas

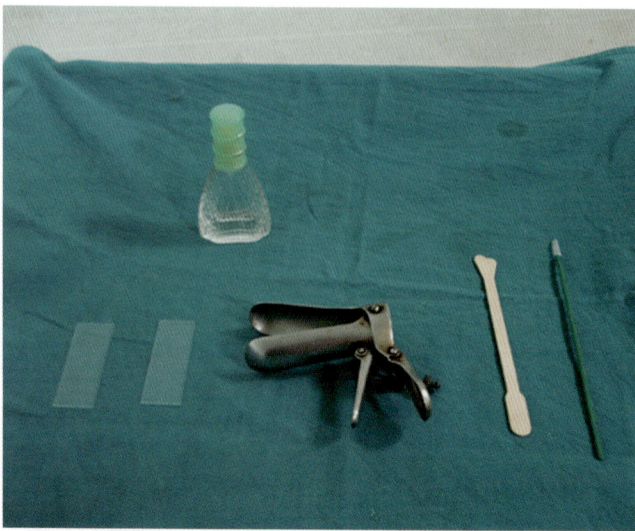

Figure 8-1: Required supplies for Pap smear

Screening Tests for Cervical Carcinoma

- Ayres wooden spatula is used commonly to sample the ectocervix.
- Endocervical brush is useful in postmenopausal women and also in those who have undergone treatment to the cervix. In these situations, the SCJ recedes inside the endocervical canal; therefore, endocervical brush is mandatory to sample the TZ. Also, in liquid-based cytology, endocervical brush is used.
- Using both Ayre's spatula and endocervical brush together will provide adequate cellularity and endocervical component and is more likely to provide satisfactory smears for interpretation.
- The endocervical broom—the Aylesbury spatula will simultaneously sample both endocervix and ectocervix **(Figure 8-2)**.
- Use of cotton swab.

The use of cotton tip applicator is not recommended. By trapping of material in the cotton fibers, it usually provides less cellular samples.[24]

Taking Pap Smear

- Before taking Pap smear, the subject should be explained how a Pap smear is taken. Label the frosted end of the glass slide with the patient's name prior to collection. With the subject in the dorsal position, the cervix is exposed adequately using a Cusco's bivalve speculum. If there is difficulty in inserting the speculum, use normal saline to moisten the surface.
- Lubrication of the vaginal introitus and speculum does not affect Papanicolaou smears.[25]
- Do not use an antiseptic solution to clean the vagina and the cervix.
- After inserting the speculum, visualize the cervix for abnormalities. The procedure should sample the squamous epithelium, columnar epithelium and the transformation zone. The TZ should be identified and sampled adequately where majority of cervical neoplasia arise. The location and appearance of the TZ are variable depending on the vaginal PH, pregnancy, hormonal mileu (age), individual anatomy and previous treatment.
- Use of moistened Ayre's spatula and endocervical brush will assist in preventing air-drying artifact.
- The Ayre's spatula is fitted to the cervical os with the long end into the endocervix. Rotate the spatula through 360° about the circumference of the cervix, in the same direction. Throughout the procedure, maintain firm contact with the epithelial surface, so that the entire SCJ is sampled **(Figures 8-3A and B)**.
- The sample is spread on a glass slide with single stroke using moderate pressure to thin out clumps of cells and mucus to get a monolayer. Excessive force will damage the cells. Both sides of the spatula should be smeared on the slide. However, as the spatula is removed, majority of material is retained on the upper horizontal surface.
- To avoid air drying and degeneration and to minimize clumping, the slide must be fixed quickly by immersing within 1–2 seconds in Coplin jar containing fixative of

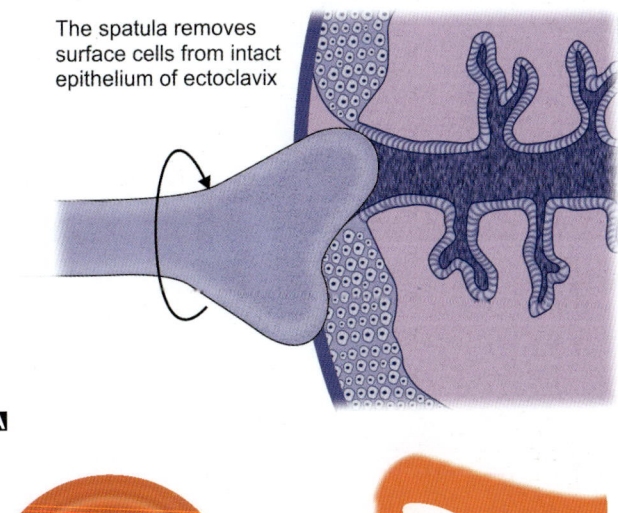

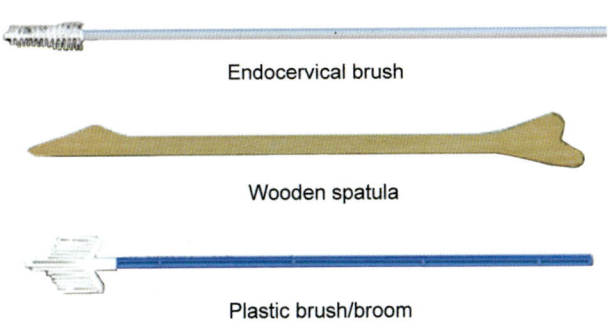

Figure 8-2: Various sampling devices

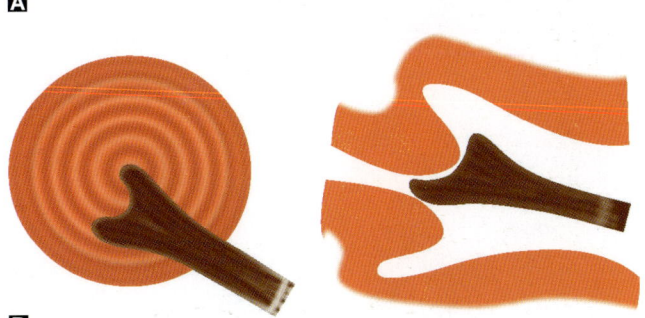

Figures 8-3A and B: Sampling of TZ with Ayre's spatula

95% ethanol or equal portion of ether and 95% ethanol or the slide can be spray fixed.

Use of Endocervical Brush (Figures 8-4A and B)

- The endocervical brush has circumferential bristles that come into contact with the entire endocervical surface
- The brush should be inserted along the axis of the cervix. If inserted at an angle to the endocervical canal, delicate endocervical stroma will be traumatized and will cause bleeding
- The brush is rotated through 180 degrees, maintaining contact with the endocervical canal **(Figures 8-4A and B)**
- Rotating the brush more than 180 degrees increases the likelihood of bleeding
- The sample is unrolled onto the slide in the opposite direction from which it was collected by twirling the brush handle **(Figure 8-5)**

- Blood may often be seen in endocervical brush sample, but rarely interferes with interpretation
- During pregnancy, use of endocervical brush is best avoided as it can trigger bleeding. Moreover, in pregnancy as the endocervix is exposed, use of Ayre's spatula can adequately sample the TZ
- Using both Ayre's spatula and endocervical brush together will provide adequate cellularity and endocervical component and is more likely to provide satisfactory smear for interpretation
- The quality of the smear can be improved by using the spatula first, followed by the endocervical brush. Using the endocervical brush first may cause bleeding from the endocervical canal and the subsequent smears will be obscured by blood.

Use of Plastic Broom (Figures 8-6A and B)

To use the 'broom', insert the long central bristles into the os until the lateral bristles bend against the ectocervix. Rotate 3–5 times in both the directions. To transfer the material, stroke both the sides of the 'broom' across the glass slide. Place the second stroke exactly over the first stroke.

EVALUATION OF CONVENTIONAL PAP SMEAR

Pap smear screening has been effective in places where the coverage and the quality of services are high and where Pap test can be done at regular intervals. A meta-analysis of the Pap test accuracy involving 62 studies comparing Pap test with histology reported that sensitivity of Pap test ranged from 11 to 99% and specificity from 14 to 97%.[26]

The Agency for Health Care Policy and Research (AHCPR), based on a meta-analysis of 84 studies, reported that conventional cytology has a specificity of 98% and a sensitivity of 51% (95% CI: 0.37–0.66). The Pap test is more

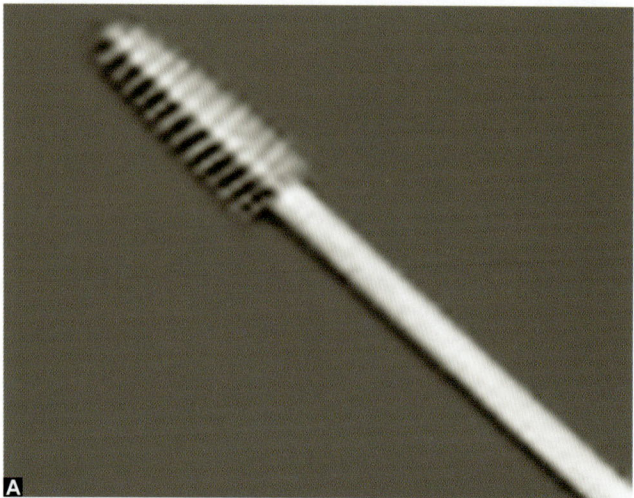
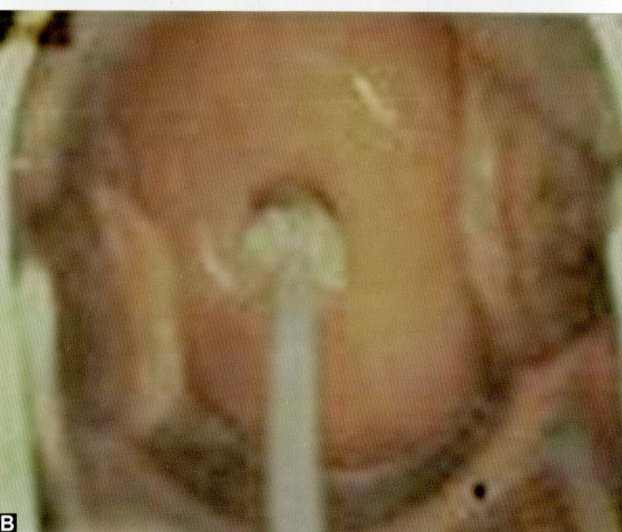

Figures 8-4A and B: Use of endocervical brush

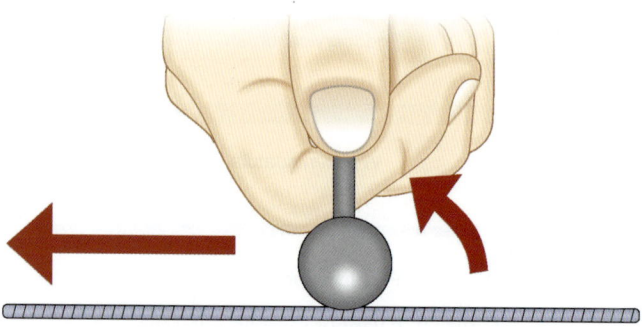

Figure 8-5: Preparing smear with endocervical brush

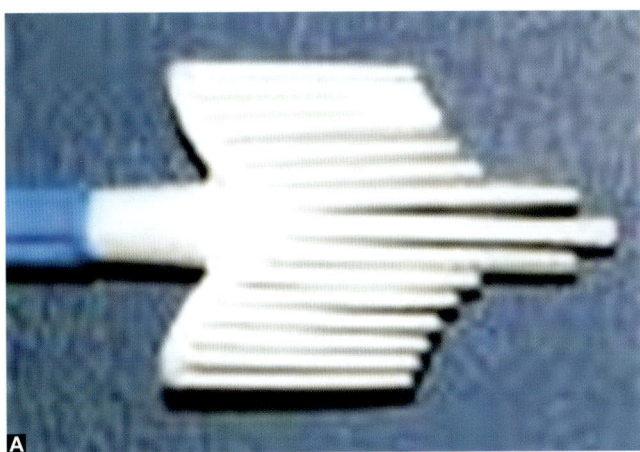
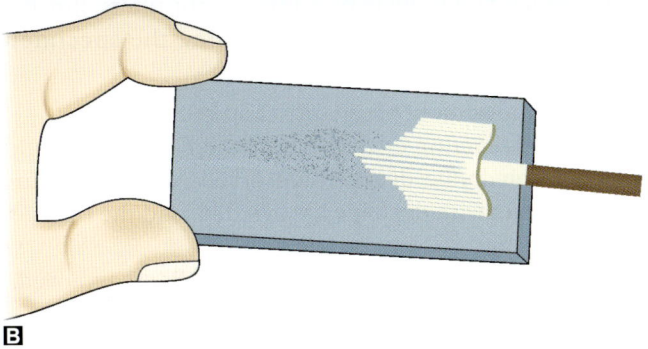

Figures 8-6A and B: Use of plastic broom

accurate when a higher cytological threshold (HSIL) is used with a goal of detecting a high-grade lesion. Lower thresholds or the use of the Pap test for detecting low-grade dysplasia results in poor discrimination.[27]

The Pap test is generally reliable in identifying women who do not have precancer and the reported false positive rate of cytology in less than 1%. However, the test misses some women who do have abnormal cells. Studies have shown that only 20% to 50% of women with precancer are correctly identified and the false negative rates are high.[26,28]

The Major Causes of False-negative Results are:

a. Inadequate Sampling

This may be due to:
- Small lesions
- Lesions eccentric on the cervix
- Lesions high in the endocervical canal
- Scarring of the cervix where TZ is difficult to sample.

b. Inappropriate Sample Technique

Studies have shown that conventional Pap smear collects from 60,000 to 1.2 million cervical epithelial cells, but less that 20% of these collected cells are transferred onto the glass slide. If the TZ is not adequately sampled, the collected cells and the transferred cells onto the slide will be few; therefore, the possibility of missing abnormal cells would be high.

In postmenopausal women, local estrogen cream may be used for 2–3 weeks to improve the cell collection.

c. Errors in Interpretation

- If the smear is too thin or too thick, the interpretation may be difficult.
- Thick areas of the overlapping epithelial cells may be seen if the samples are taken in the late luteal phase. Therefore, Pap smear should be taken preferably in the first half of the cycle.
- In the presence of obvious infection, cells will be obscured. Therefore, infection should be treated before taking a Pap smear.
- As RBCs can also obscure the fields, Pap smear should not be taken closer to periods.
- It is important to fix the slides immediately as air drying can cause degeneration of cells.
- Cells from necrotic areas may not be recognizable.
- Good staining technique is also important, as interpretation may be difficult with poor staining techniques.

d. Professional Error

Cytology requires intense microscopic review of cells. Therefore, professional errors can occur due to inexperience, or due to intensity of work. Quality assurance studies indicate that even skilled screening cytologists can have a false negative fraction of 5%.

> - 2/3rds of false negatives are due to inadequate sampling, sample transfers and preparation errors
> - 1/3rd of false negatives are due to interpretation errors.

LIQUID-BASED THIN-LAYER CYTOLOGY (LBC)

The aim of fluid-based technology (monolayer) is to reduce the incidence of false negative cytological findings by optimizing the collection and preparation of cells.

Two systems are available which create a monolayer for cervical cytological studies.
- Thinprep. Cytyc Corporation, Boxborough, Maes.
- CytoRich, Roche Image Analysis Systems, Inc. Elan College, NC

The sensitivity of the conventional Pap smear for the detection of cervical cancer precursor is less than 50%. The major limitations posed by the conventional Pap smear are:

1. Only 20% of the collected cells are transferred to the slide.
2. Inadequate fixation due to air drying resulting in artifacts and degeneration of cells.
3. The abnormal cells are randomly distributed.
4. There are obscuring elements, such as blood, mucus and inflammatory cells.

In order to overcome the above limitations liquid-based thin layer technology was introduced. Thin layer slides prepared in this system reduce the obscuring features, also there is improved cell transfer from the collecting device to the slide.

Method of Collecting and Processing of Sample

In LBC, the cervical cells are collected using a cytobrush or a broom. The cervical collection device is immersed into the liquid fixative and rinsed. This allows mechanical mixing and homogenous distribution of cells in the solution **(Figure 8-7)**.

The device contains a polycarbonate cylinder that holds a membrane with an 8 μ pore size. As the collected fluid passes through this semipermeable barrier, the membrane detains epithelial cells and infective organisms, but the debris and inflammatory cells are allowed to pass. The thin cellular material collected is transferred onto a glass slide spread in a circular fashion and fixed. The prepared slide can be screened manually or by automated screening techniques.

Advantages of LBC

The preservative solution has a high alcohol content, therefore, preserves cells during transport, lyses fresh red cells and kills microbiological elements. The solution preserves the morphological details of the cells, strengthens the bonds between cells in clusters limiting disaggregation, and makes the cell more rigid so that it is more difficult for them to pass through the filters. Rinsing the cells into vials and homogenizing the specimen ensures randomization.

1. The entire amount of cells are captured.
2. As the collecting device is immersed into the liquid fixative air drying, degeneration of cells, cell damage due to contract with dry slide are avoided, and the cells get fixed instantly.
3. Obscuring debris and inflammatory cells are removed.
4. Thin layers of cells are produced.
5. There is uniform distribution of abnormal cells, if present.
6. There is no selective loss of small abnormal cells.
7. The remaining fluid in the vial can be used for HPV DNA triage or to perform tests for *Neisseria gonorrhoea* or HPV or *Chlamydia trachomatis*.
8. This technology removes most mucus, protein and fresh red blood cells, distributes the cells uniformly, improves fixation and preservation of cellular structure, maintains diagnostic clusters and ensures uniform sampling of the material removed from the cervix.

The prepared slide contains 50,000–75,000 cells per slide in circular areas.

Limitations of LBC

- It is more expensive and needs special instrumentation than conventional cytology.
- Interpretation of monolayer is difficult from conventional cytological studies, requires retraining of cytotechnologists and cytopathologists.
- Nuclear size is smaller and chromatin is more evenly distributed. At low magnification, such groups of cells may be overlooked because they resemble metaplastic cells.
- Also, glandular abnormalities are more difficult to assess because the cell clusters remain spherical in thin layers rather than being flattened as in conventional smears.

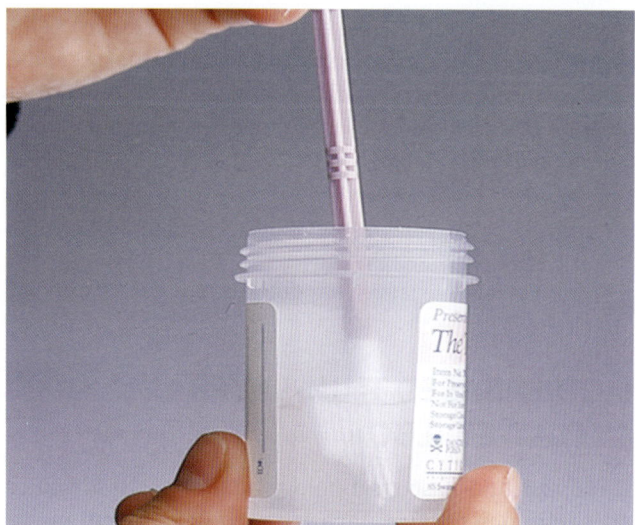

Figure 8-7: Collection of cells in LBC

Automated Screening Technology

For an effective cervical cancer screening program, the false-negative and false-positive results of cytology should be kept minimum. Manual screening of cytology slides is labor intensive and difficult, because the technician has to identify a few abnormal cells among thousands of normal cells.[29]

Moreover, the screening process is subjective and there is always inter and intraobserver variation. In order to reduce the workload and to reduce diagnostic errors, automated screening techniques have been developed. By using these techniques, false-negative Pap test results are also reduced. With these methods not only the primary screening of cervical smears, but also, quality control rescreening can be done.

The automated screening techniques rely on neural network technology and are based on computerized imaging and identification of abnormal cervical cells. These techniques necessitate collection of cytology specimen in a liquid-based medium and processing in an automated preparation system so as to have a thin layer of cells.

Two automated systems are approved by FDA-USA.
- PAPNET Testing System (Neuromedical System, Inc., Suffern, NY)
- Neopath Auto Pap 300 QC System (Neopath, Inc., Redmont, WA).

PAPNET[30,31]

The PAPNET 19 is a semiautomated system, which consists of two phases, a scanning phase and a review phase for cervical smears. The Thin Prep imaging system scans the slides and identifies 22 fields most likely to contain abnormal cells and these images are stored. These stored images are then viewed by a trained cytologist and triaged as either 'negative' or review. The slides that are placed in the 'review' category are screened manually. Later, a pathologist reviews the abnormal slide to determine the final diagnosis.

Studies have shown that screening with PAPNET is more likely to identify potentially abnormal cells than manual screening.

Neopath AutoPap 300 QC System:[32] (also known as Focal Point™ System)

In this technique, the prepared cervical smears are affixed with a barcode and loaded into trays and placed into the slide processor, which first reads the barcode, checks each slide for physical integrity, then scans and analyzes the slide. The system utilizes specialized, computerized high-speed video-microscope and image interpretation software. During scanning, each slide is analyzed for specimen adequacy and morphological changes indicative of epithelial abnormalities. The slide is then assigned a score based on the likelihood that the individual slide is benign, unsatisfactory or abnormal. The cells are then classified into those requiring 'no review' and those requiring 'review'. The abnormal slides are reviewed manually by the cytopathologist. On evaluating Auto Pap system and Manual screening, automated screening was found to be more sensitive in identifying ASCUS and LSIL and equivalent to manual screening for the detection of HSIL.

EFFICACY OF LIQUID-BASED CYTOLOGY

LBC enhances both the nuclear irregularities and the chromosomal pattern and highlights the cytoplasmic cavity enhancing the true internal border of Koilocytic cells.

Ronco et al. (2000), recruited 45,000 women (aged 25-60 years) to undergo cancer screening with either conventional or LBC. The study concluded that compared with conventional cytology, LBC predicted more mild abnormalities and reduced the number of unsatisfactory smears. It also allows reflex testing for HPV. However, unlike its higher sensitivity for detecting CIN Grade I lesions, its sensitivity for detecting high-grade CIN was similar to that of conventional cytology.[33]

Davey et al. (2004-2005) compared the accuracy of LBC using computer assistance with that of manually read conventional cytology. With thin Prep Imager, significantly fewer slides were found to be unsatisfactory for examination than with manual reading (1.8% vs 3.1%) and significantly more low-grade and high-grade histologic abnormalities were found with Thin Prep Imager than with manual reading. Thin Prep Imager also was significantly less likely to classify slides as 'Inconclusive', high-grade lesions to be excluded (ASC-H).[34]

FREQUENCY OF PAP SMEAR TESTING

Recommendations for initiation and frequency of cervical cancer screening vary from country to country. Studies have shown that increased frequency of cytological sampling can result in greater reduction in the cumulative rate of invasive carcinoma **(Table 8.2)**.

Based on the evidence published in 2003, the NHS (UK) (National Health Service), cervical cancer screening programe now offers screening at different intervals depending on age.[35]

In the UK, screening is initiated at the age of 25 years. It had been shown that under the age of 25 years, invasive cancer is extremely rare but changes in the cervix are common and most lesions would regress. Therefore, screening women less than 25 years of age would result in unnecessary investigation and treatment. The screening

Table 8-2: Percentage reduction in cumulative rate of invasive cervical cancer with different frequency of screening	
Screening frequency in years	Reduction in cumulative rate %
1	93.3%
2	92.5%
3	91.4%
5	83.9%
10	64.2%

[Data from IARC working group. Screening for cancer of the uterine cervix. Lyon France, International Agency for Research on Cancer, 1986 P (4)]

Table 8-3: Screening guidelines by various organizations			
Guideline	NHS UK-2003	American Cancer Society, 2002	American College of Obstetricians and Gynecologists 2003
Initial screening	25 years	Age 21 or 3 years after vaginal sex	Age 21 or 3 years after vaginal sex
Interval	25–49 years 3 yearly 50–65 years 5 yearly	Upto 30 years Every year for conventional Pap Every 2 years for LBC After 30 years Every 2–3 years if 3 consecutive tests were negative	Upto 30 years Every year for either LBC or conventional cytology After 30 years Every 2–3 years if 3 consecutive tests were negative
Discontinue	65 years with previous 3 negative tests	70 years with 3 consecutive normal in 10 years	No upper limit of age

is discontinued at the age of 65 years; because it is unlikely that such women will go on to develop the disease if the previous smears had been negative. However, women who have not been screened since the age of 50 or have had recent abnormal tests are continued to be screened.

The American Cancer Society (ACS) and American College of Obstetricians and Gynecologists (ACOG) advocate early initiation of screening, more frequent testing and continue screening until 70 years of age and above. The screening is discontinued at the age of 70, who had at least three documented consecutive normal cervical cytology and no abnormal tests in the previous 10 years. However, women who have had a history of cervical carcinoma, in-utero exposure to DES and women, who are immunocompromised, should continue cervical cancer screening as long as they are in good healt (Table 8-3).[36]

In women with the following high risk factors, even after the age of 30 years more frequent screening is required.
1. HIV positive women
2. Immunocompromised patients by organ transplant, chemotherapy, chronic corticosteroid treatment
3. Those with prior CIN2/3
4. Previous DES exposure.

POST HYSTERECTOMY

Post hysterectomy Smear

- Majority of evidence suggests that women who have had a total hysterectomy for benign disease do not need further Pap smear testing, provided the cervix is completely removed and previous Pap smears were normal.
- In women, who have had supracervical hysterectomy, screening, should be done as per the guidelines.
- In women who have had previous abnormal smears or hysterectomy was done for CIN2/CIN3.
- Repeat vault smear at 6 moths and 12 months respectively.
- If both are negative, discontinue all vault smears.
- If vault smears are positive and if there is suspicion that premalignant condition is not completely removed, continue with annual vault smears.

Chapter 9

HPV DNA Testing

By strong epidemiological, clinical and molecular studies it has been shown that infection of the cervix with high-risk HPV is a necessary early event in cervical carcinogenesis. The association between infection with high-risk HPV and high-grade CIN lesion and cervical cancer is so strong that HPV DNA testing has been explored as a disease marker by various studies throughout the world.

While using HPV DNA testing, the following facts should be taken into consideration:[37]

- Most infections in young women are transient
- Transient HPV infections are much less common in women older than 30 years than among young women
- HPV DNA positivity drops after the age of 30 years. Peak levels of HPV high-risk types occur in 20–25% of women between 20 and 24 years. For those over the age of 35 years, persistent high-risk types are seen in only 4–5% of cases.

> Therefore, in settings where only 1 to 3 screens can be performed in a woman's lifetime, screening by HPV DNA testing should not be initiated before the age of 30–35 years

ADVANTAGES OF HPV DNA TESTING AS A SCREENING TEST[38]

Compared with cytological evaluation or visual inspection of the cervix:

1. The test has high sensitivity. This is important in settings where women will be screened only once or twice in their lifetime.
2. HPV DNA testing not only identifies women with cervical disease but also those who are at risk of developing cervical neoplasia within the next 3 to 10 years. The presence of DNA for high-risk HPV types (even in the presence of negative cytology) identified women who are at risk of progressing to disease. This will have importance for developing countries where sufficient resources will not be available to screen women at frequent intervals.
3. The interpretation of HPV DNA testing is objective and does not have the inherent subjectivity of visual screening methods or cervical cytological assessment.

Clinical Uses of HPV DNA Testing

1. IN THE MANAGEMENT OF MILDLY ABNORMAL SMEARS:

> - In UK, cervical screening program
>   Borderline changes and mild dyskaryosis
> - In Bethesda classification
>   ASC-US and LSIL

There has been a controversy in the management of low-grade cytological abnormalities. This is because of the findings that 5–20% of women with low-grade cytological findings (ASC-US or LSIL) may harbor undetected high-grade lesions. In order to detect those with high-grade lesions, the options available are immediate colposcopy or repeated cytologic assessment at 6–12-month intervals. Both these methods may require repeated clinic visits.

HPV–DNA Triage

Now it has been shown that in women of all ages, when the Pap smear indicates ASC–US or borderline changes, HPV

DNA testing will help the clinician in management decision. This is called HPV DNA triage. (The term 'triaging' is commonly used to mean sorting low- from high-risk women).

Those women who are test positive for high-risk HPV types are followed more closely, and colposcopy performed than those who are test negative. Manos et al. undertook secondary screening of women who had the so-called ASC-US smears using repeated cytology, colposcopy and HPV testing. The key findings were that when the HPV testing was negative high-grade CIN lesions were negative. Therefore, it is valuable in identifying women in whom colposcopy is not required (high negative predictive value). Testing positive does not mean that there is an underlying disease, but, indicates that close follow-up and further evaluation are necessary. HPV detection in older women is likely to represent persistent infection and persistence is predictive of disease detection. The positive predictive value of HPV DNA for the detection of CIN rises with age.[39]

The ASC-US/LSIL Triage Study (ALTS) Trial

This is a large randomized trial specifically designed to evaluate three methods of managing women with cytologic findings with ASC-US and LSIL.

The three methods compared were:
1. Immediate colposcopic examination for all women.
2. HPV testing and referral for colposcopy if HPV test result was positive.
3. Repeated cytologic assessment with referral for colposcopy if the smear showed the presence of HSIL.

The findings were as follows:
- Approximately 80% of the women who had a cytologic diagnosis of LSIL were found to harbor HPV DNA.
- Because vast majority of women with LSIL tested positive for HPV, HPV testing had no value as a triaging agent.

> HPV testing is not of value in the management of women found to have LSIL on cytological evaluation.
> *ALTS Trial*
>
> **Recommendation:**
> Women with LSIL on cytological evaluation should undergo colposcopy instead of HPV testing.   *ASCCP*

With regard to the management of women found to have ASC-US, the ALTS trial found that HPV testing detected 96.3% of women with previously undiagnosed CIN3 or cancer and resulted in the referral of only 56.1% of women for colposcopy. This would significantly reduce the number of women requiring colposcopy. If LBC was used for the initial cervical smear, then reflex HPV testing (that is using the residual fluid in the LBC sample for HPV testing, if the cytologic diagnosis is ASC-US) is the preferred option. And this will make the second clinic visit unnecessary.[40]

2. HPV DNA Testing for Post-treatment Follow-up of CIN Lesions

Ablative or excisional methods for the treatment of CIN lesion are very effective and more than 90% of cure rate has been reported. However, in 5% to 15% of cases, the precursor lesion will persist or recur requiring close follow-up and retreatment. A combination of cytologic and Colposcopic assessment has been used to follow-up these women post treatment. Based on the fact that without detectable HPV, the likelihood of post-treatment persistence or recurrence of disease is negligible. HPV DNA testing has recently been investigated as an alternative to these two diagnostic modalities. Studies so far have suggested that HPV testing may be significantly more reliable than colposcopy and cytology.[41]

3. HPV DNA Testing as a Primary Screening Test

Several studies have demonstrated the value of testing for HPV DNA in primary screening.
- In women more than 35 years of age, HPV DNA testing is used as a primary screening tool as an adjunct to cytology. High-risk HPV types in women above 35 years are likely to reflect persistent high-risk infection, which can progress to invasive cervical carcinoma.
- Even if the cytology is reported normal, positive HPV testing will identify women with disease or those at risk of disease.
- WHO recommendations now include HPV testing as an acceptable method of primary screening for cervical cancer prevention.

In 2003, the US Food and Drug administration approved HPV DNA testing combined with cervical cytology as a screening technique for women older than 30 years. When the results of both the tests are negative, the woman does not have to be retested.[42] The negative predictive value of a double negative test exceeds 99%.[43]

4. Clarification of Noncorrelating Colposcopy

When colposcopy examination fails to detect the source of an abnormal Pap test, HPV testing helps to resolve these conflicting results.

5. Test of Cure

HPV testing following treatment can be used to ensure both disease and HPV have been eradicated.

Limitations of HPV DNA Testing

- The testing requires expensive laboratory technology and special computers. In developing countries like India, there will be financial constraints in using this technology
- It is labor-intensive for mass screening
- HPV positive testing has a very high sensitivity to detect high-grade CIN lesions. However, the specificity is relatively poor, particularly in younger women in whom the infection is common. Therefore, HPV DNA testing for mass screening will identify more positive cases in young women, in whom the infection is transient.

Diagnosis of HPV Infection

The diagnosis of HPV infection can be made from clinical findings, morphologic, serologic and molecular biology techniques.
- Clinical diagnosis of HPV infection can be made by the presence of warty lesions in the cervix, vagina and perianal regions
- Morphologically, HPV infection can be demonstrated in cytological smears and biopsy specimens. In productive infections such as warts, virus particles about 50 nm in diameter can be detected by electron microscopy
- Immunological detection of HPV in human tissue is limited by various reasons:
    a. The late capsid proteins (L1, L2) are expressed only in productive infections
    b. The early proteins E6 or E7 are often expressed in low amounts in the infected tissues
    c. And there is lack of sensitive, specific antibodies against the viral proteins.

Molecular Biology Techniques

As HPV cannot be propagated in tissue culture, molecular biology techniques are used for its identification. The molecular diagnosis of HPV in clinical specimen is based on nucleic acid probe technology. Direct detection of HPV genomes as well as transcripts can be achieved with hybridization procedures that include Southern and Northern blots, dot blots, in-situ hybridization and signal, and amplification molecular technology.

Presently, two assays are widely used for the detection of genital types, namely:
1. Digene Hybrid Capture assay, version hc2.
2. PCR with generic primers.

Hybrid Capture Assays *(Version hc2: Digene, Gaithersburg, MD, USA)*

This assay uses signal amplification molecular technology and is based on hybridization, where synthetic RNA probes are used. There are two probes, namely A probe and B probe.

The 'A' probe cocktail has RNA probes to detect 5 low-risk types of HPV. namely 6, 11, 42, 43 and 44.

The 'B' probe cocktail has RNA probe to detect 13 high-risk types of HPV in two separate reactions (types 16, 18, 31, 33, 35, 39, 45, 51, 52, 56, 58, 59 and 68).

Methodology

Specific HPV DNA-RNA hybrids are formed in solution and then captured by antibodies. The immobilized hybrids are detected by a series of reactions that generate a luminescent product that can be measured in a luminometer. The intensity of emitted light, expressed as relative light units (RLUs) is proportional to the amount of target DNA present in the specimen.

The US Food and Drug Administration recommended the cut-off value for test-positive results to be 1.0 RLU (equivalent to 1 pg of HPV DNA per 1 mL of sampling buffer).

The technique is easy to perform in clinical setting, does not require special facilities to avoid cross contamination and does not require amplification target to be highly sensitive.

However, this assay identifies high-risk HPV types in a group and can not discriminate between individual types.[38,44]

PCR-based Assay for HPV Detection and Typing

The only procedure that may be capable of recognizing all HPV types and variants present in a biologic specimen is DNA sequencing of the viral genome, either after cloning into plasmids or by direct sequencing of a polymerase chain reaction (PCR) fragment. PCR technique is based on target amplification. PCR can produce one billion copies from a single double-stranded DNA molecule after 30 cycles of amplification. Therefore, care must be taken to avoid false-positive results derived from cross-contaminant specimens or reagents. The most widely used PCR protocols use consensus primers directed to a highly conserved region of the L1 gene and have the potential to detect all mucosal HPV types. Primers such as GP 5/6, and the MY 09/11 are widely used. Unlike Hybrid Capture Assay, PCR-based methods can discriminate between individual HPV types. Both the techniques can provide viral load information.[44]

Chapter 10

Cytology of Normal and Abnormal Cells of Cervix

NORMAL CYTOLOGY

The stratified squamous cells are markedly cohesive. Therefore, cells removed from the ectocervix are those that have exfoliated from the surface. Under microscopy, they are seen as individual cells. The columnar cells are less cohesive and can be removed in clumps.

In the well-estrogenized women, majority of squamous cells are from the superficial and intermediate layers. These cells are navicular in shape, have abundant cytoplasm, the nuclei are round, small and centrally located **(Figure 10-1)**.

When columnar cells are present, they appear linear in arrangement with basal nuclei and grouped in a honeycomb pattern **(Figure 10-2)**.

The amount of cells that are exfoliated varies with the menstrual cycle. During the proliferative phase, there is increased exfoliation of well-glycogenated superficial cells. However, in the secretary phase, the predominant cells are intermediate and the cells have less glycogen. In the postmenopausal women, the exfoliated cells are mostly parabasal with some intermediate forms. These cells are smaller in size, and more rounded with large centrally located nuclei.

The nuclear membrane in normal cells is smooth, and the nuclear chromatin is usually granular and finely stippled.

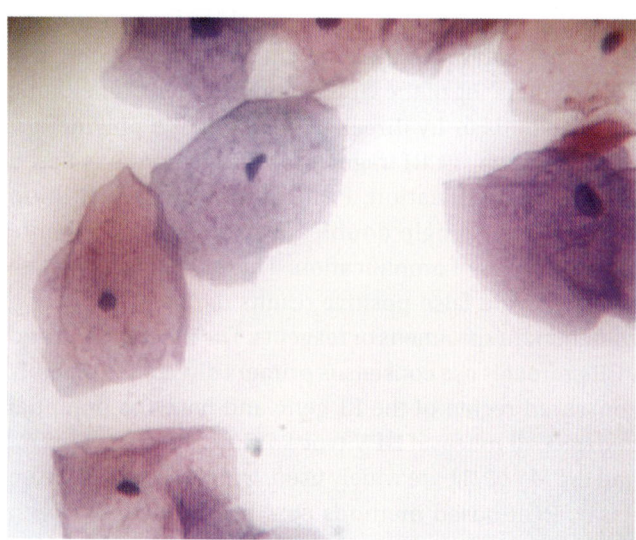

Figure 10-1: The normal squamous cells

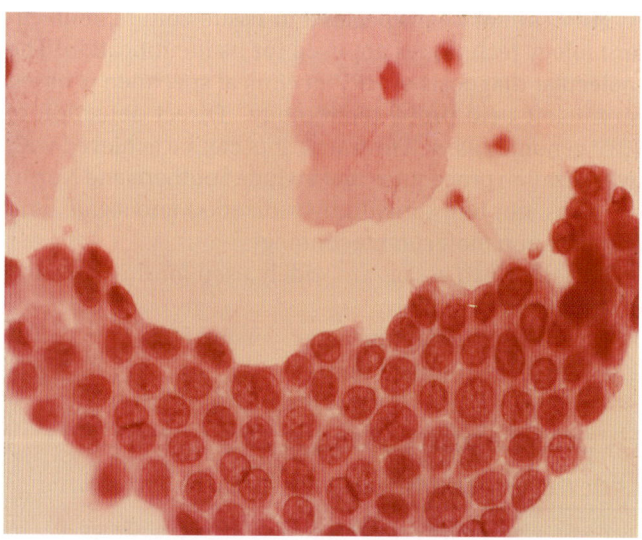

Figure 10-2: The normal endocervical cells

Inflammatory Smear (Figure 10-3)

In inflammatory smears, the entire field is covered with pus cells masking the details of the squamous cells. Therefore, with inflammatory smear reports, infection should be treated and smear should be repeated.

Atypical Squamous Cells of Undetermined Significance (ASC-US) (Figures 10-4A and B)

Here a distinction between reactive and neoplastic cells cannot be made by the cytopathologist. The nuclei of these cells are enlarged 2–3 times more than a normal intermediate cell. As a result, the nucleus to cytoplasmic ratio is increased and the chromatin content is more (hyperchromasia). However, there is absence of nuclear irregularities to call it abnormal.

Atypical Squamous Cells of Undetermined Significance Cannot Exclude HSIL

Here the nuclear atypia is seen in immature squamous metaplastic cells. The nuclei are enlarged 2–3 times above the normal metaplastic cells, resulting in increased nucleus cytoplasmic ratio, increased chromatin content, variations in nuclear size and shape, and nuclear membrane irregularity.

The Cytology of Low-grade Squamous Intraepithelial Lesion (LSIL) (Figures 10-5A and B)

Here the atypia is seen in mature cells. The abnormal squamous cells are equivalent in size to a normal superficial or intermediate cells. There is enlargement of the nucleus, 2-3 times the normal, increase in chromatin content and irregularity in chromatin distribution. The size and shape of nucleus vary with binucleation and multinucleation **(Figure 10-6)**. The nuclear membrane is irregular. There may be cavitation of cytoplasm, immediately surrounding the nucleus to form a well-demarcated internal cytoplasmic border, the perinuclear halo. This is referred to as koilocytosis. In the absence of nuclear features, koilocytosis should not be coined as LSIL. The squamous epithelium frequently becomes acanthotic (or thickened) (Perinuclear

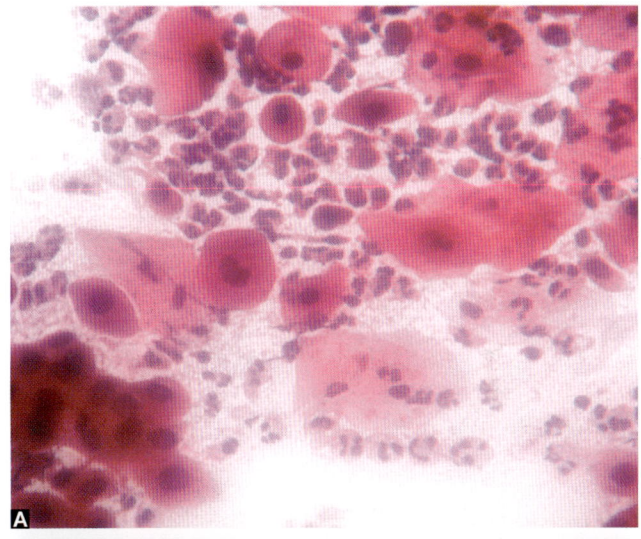

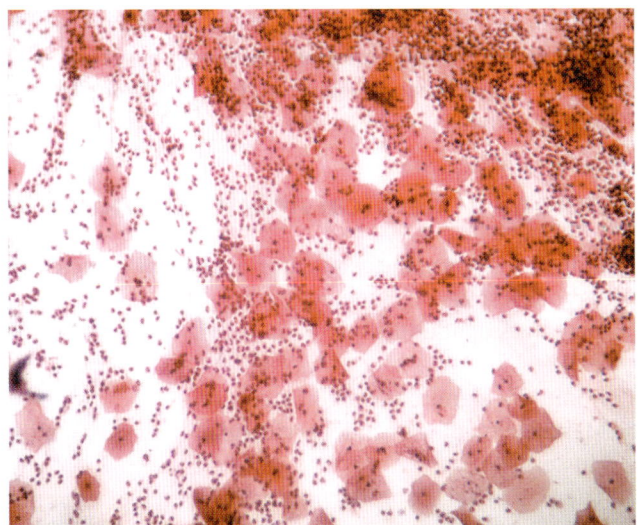

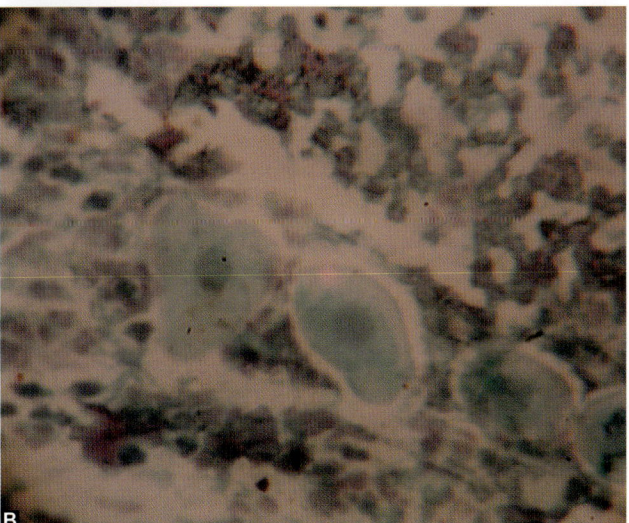

Figure 10-3: Inflammatory smears

Figures 10-4A and B: (A) ASC-US; (B) Pap stain—high power magnification—ASC-US

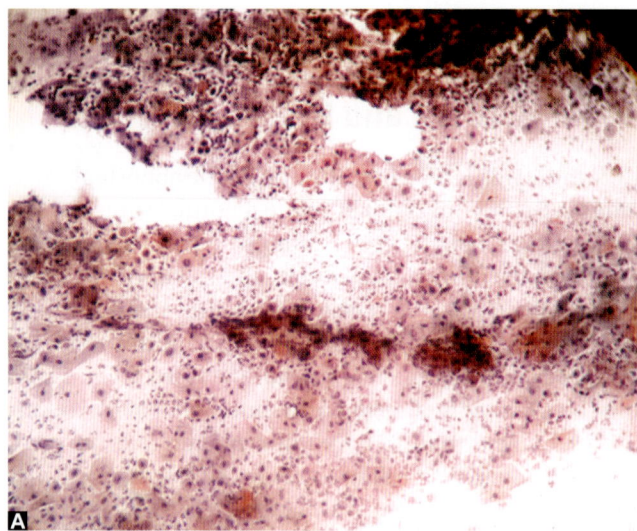

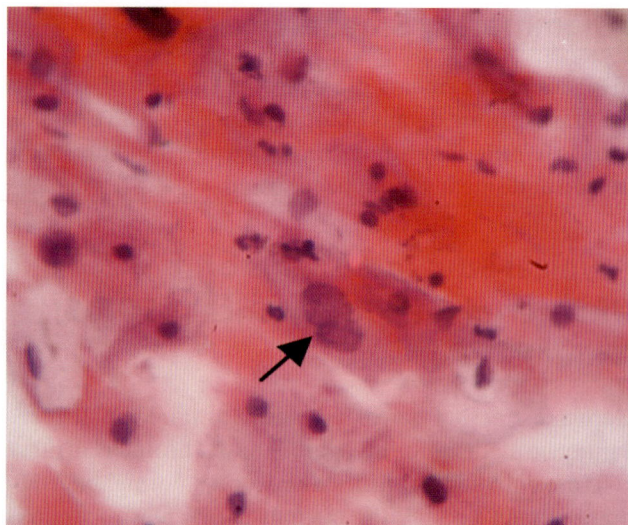

Figure 10-6: Binuclear cells in LSIL

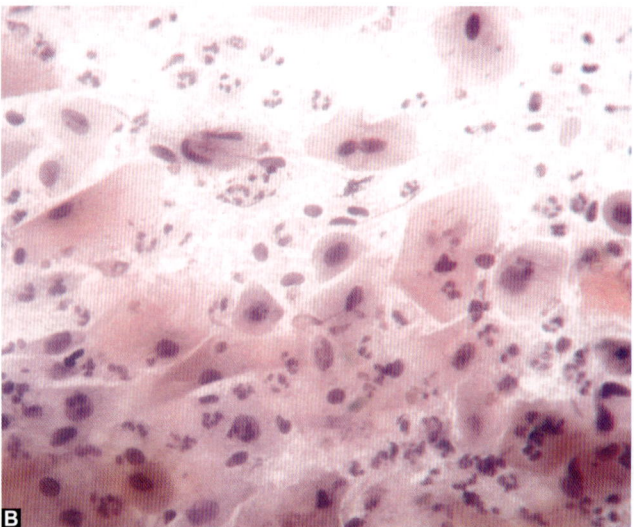

Figures 10-5A and B: Cytology of LSIL

There is nuclear enlargement, and the enlargement is the same as that of a low-grade lesion. Because of the smaller size of the cells in HSIL, there is marked increase in nuclear to cytoplasmic ratio. Sometimes, only a very thin rim of cytoplasm is seen around the nucleus, making it more prominent, referred to as 'naked nuclei'. There is marked irregularity of the nuclear membrane, irregular chromatin distribution, marked hyperchromasia, clumping of nuclear material and variation in nuclear size and shape. Syncytial groups are also possible.

Cytology of Squamous Cell Carcinoma (Figures 10-8A and B)

In squamous cell carcinoma, there are spindle-shaped cells, hyperchromasia, abnormal mitotic figures and tumor diathesis due to breachment of the basement membrane. Perinuclear halo is seen in some of the cells.

Cytology of Cervical Adenocarcinoma

Glandular lesions of the cervix are not as easily detected as squamous lesions on cytology.

Diagnosis of adenocarcinoma is made by the presence of:
1. Abundant glandular cellular material
2. Marked crowding of endocervical glandular cells within clusters.
3. There is cellular atypia with marked nuclear enlargement, hyperchromasia and nuclear crowding.
4. Orderly arrangement between the cells is lost.

halo without atypia can also be seen in infections such as *Trichomonas vaginalis*, *Gardnerella vaginalis*, *Candida* infection and occasionally in postmenopausal women with squamous metaplasia). Nuclear enlargement with atypia is necessary to make the diagnosis of LSIL.

High-grade Squamous Intraepithelial Lesion (HSIL) (Figures 10-7A to F)

Here the atypia is seen in immature cells. The size of a high-grade SIL is smaller than those seen in low-grade lesions and are equivalent to that of normal parabasal cells (The cells of low-grade lesions are of the size of an intermediate cell). As they get more dysplastic, the cells get elongated.

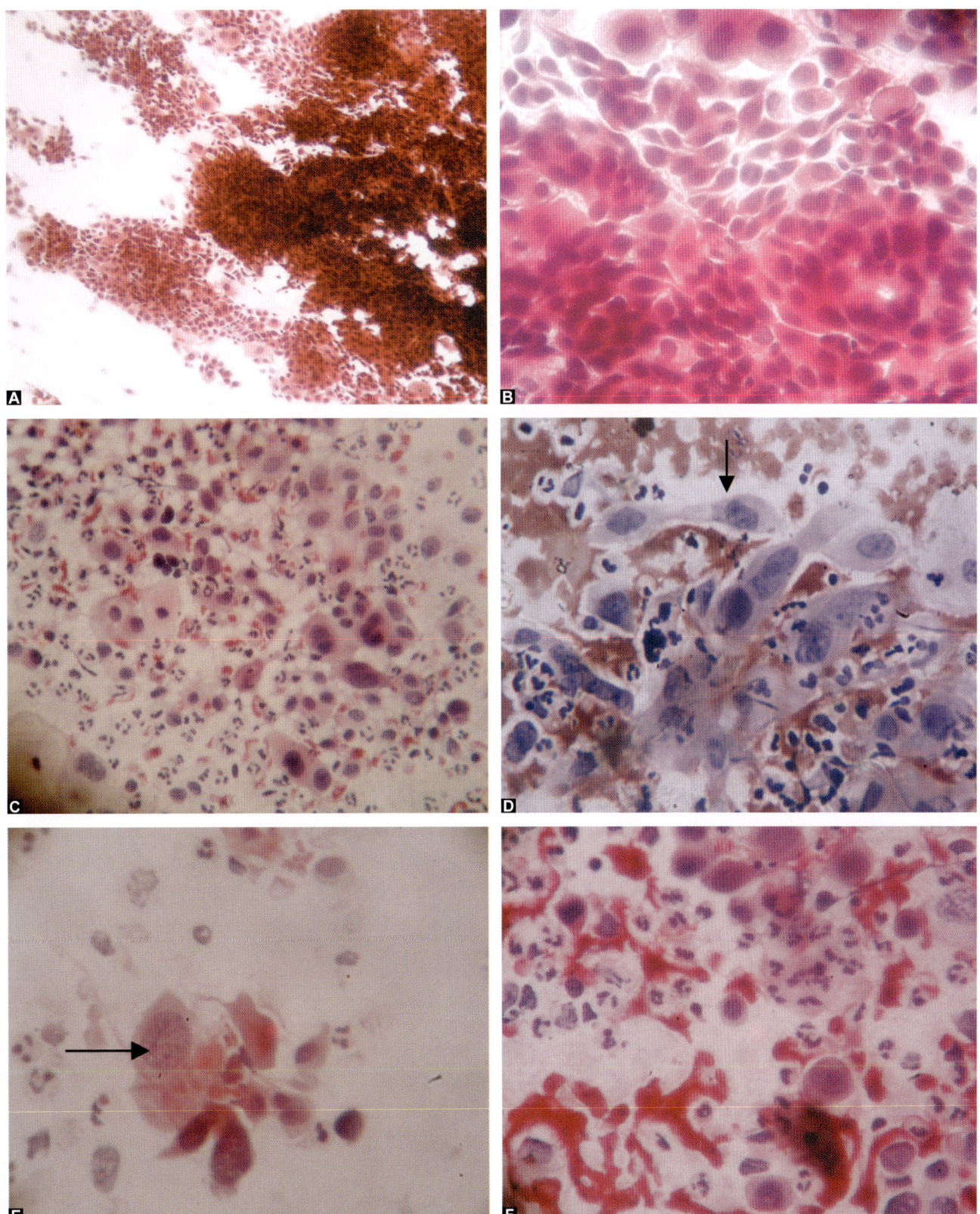

Figures 10-7A to F: Cytology pictures showing HSIL. A. Low power; B. High power; C. Picture showing tumor diathesis eliciting inflammatory reaction; D. Cells are showing irregular chromatin. Tadpole cells are also seen; E. Nucleus showing irregular chromatin; and F. HSIL-Pap stain

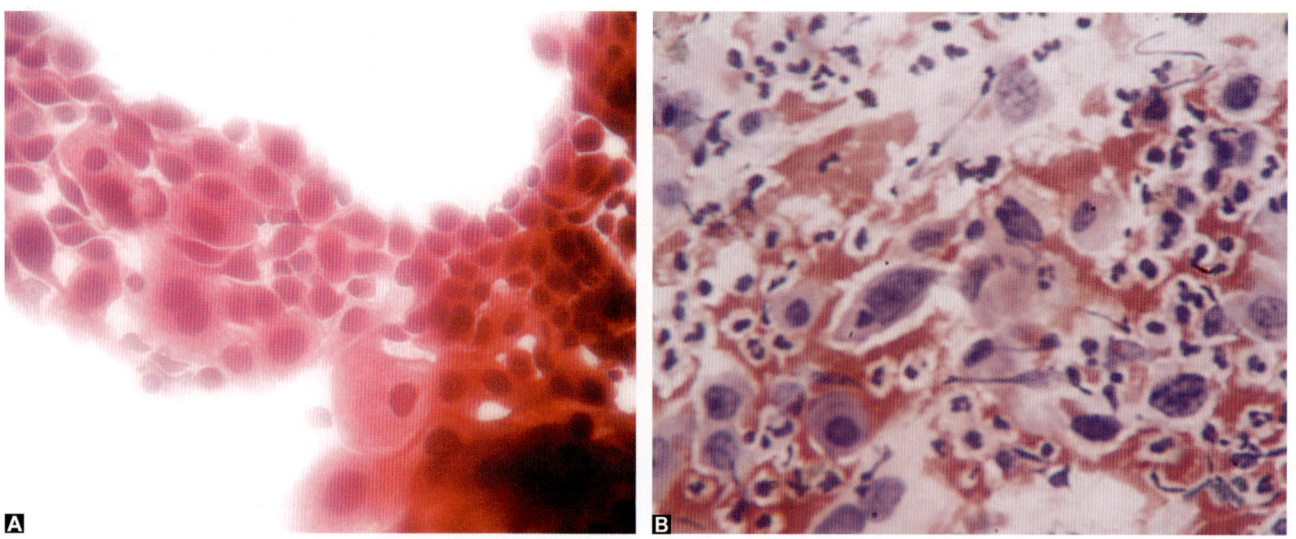

Figures 10-8A and B: A. Cytology picture showing spindle shaped cell in invasive carcinoma, B. Cytology picture showing abnormal shaped cells and breachment of the basement membrane.

Cytology Changes in Pregnancy

In the presence of high estrogen milieu of pregnancy, the cellular components of the cervix are altered. The basal cell hyperplasia, Arias-stella reaction and immature metaplasia, which occur during pregnancy, may interfere with Pap smear interpretation. However, CIN changes in pregnancy are the same as that of the nonpregnant women.

Chapter 11

Management of Abnormal Cytology Cell Results

MANAGEMENT OF ATYPICAL SQUAMOUS CELLS

Atypical squamous cells (ASCs) indicate that cytologic findings are suggestive, but not diagnostic, of a squamous intraepithelial lesion.

Atypical squamous cells are further subcategorized into:
- Atypical squamous cells of undetermined significance (ASC-US).
- Atypical squamous cells cannot exclude HSIL (ASC-H).

In the management of atypical squamous cells, several points are to be taken into consideration. Even among expert cytopathologists, a smear report of atypical squamous cells is the least reproducible.[45]

Management of ASC-US (Figure 11-1)

In the management of ASC-US, it is important to understand that the prevalence of CIN2, 3 ranges from 5–16% in women with ASC-US report.[46] However, the prevalence of invasive cancer is low in women with ASC-US (0.1–0.2%).[47]

Because of the dilemma in the management of mild cytologic abnormalities, the National Cancer Institute implemented a multicenter randomized trial. The ASC-US/LSIL Triage Study (ALTS). The ALTS study was designed to compare HPV testing, repeat cytology and colposcopy in detecting CIN3 lesions in women who have had mild cytologic abnormalities.[48,49]

Based on the ALTS study, the 2001 and 2006 consensus guidelines of ASCCP stated that testing for high-risk oncogenic HPV, repeat cytological examination at 6 months' interval or a colposcopic examination are effective approaches for managing women over the age of 20 years with ASC-US.

'Reflex' testing refers to testing either the original liquid-based cytology residual specimen or a separate sample co-collected at the time of the initial screening visit for HPV testing.

A. In women with ASC-US, whenever HPV triage is used, if the HPV DNA is negative, they are followed up with repeat cytological testing at 12 months and those women, who are HPV DNA positive, are referred for colposcopic examination.
B. When repeat cytological testing is used for managing women with ASC-US, cytological testing is preferred at 6-month intervals until two negative results are obtained. If repeat testing is consistently positive, they are referred for colposcopic examination.

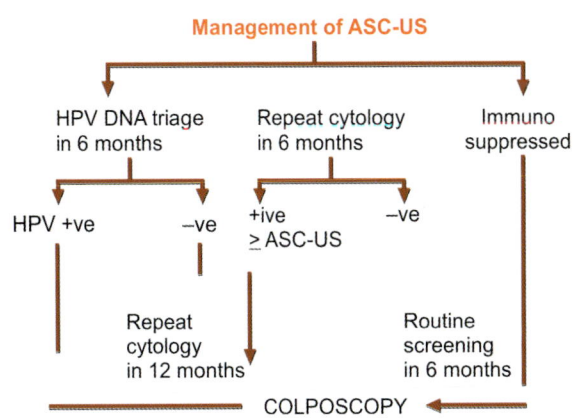

Figure 11-1: Flowchart showing management of ASC-US

C. If colposcopy is initially used to manage women with ASC-US:
   – If CIN is diagnosed, they are treated as per guidelines.
   – However, if CIN is not diagnosed at colposcopy (a single colposcopic examination can miss significant lesion), further follow-up is necessary with either HPV testing at 12 months or 2 repeat cytological examinations performed at 6 months' intervals. (It is recommended that HPV DNA testing should not be performed at intervals less than 12 months.)
D. Because of the potential for overtreatment in the absence of histologically diagnosed CIN2, 3, diagnostic excisional procedures such as LEEP (LOOP Electrosurgical Excision) is unacceptable as the initial management.
E. Those women who were followed up with HPV/ cytology, if HPV DNA is positive or cytology is persistently positive for ASC-US, they are referred for colposcopy. It is recommended that in these women, endocervical sampling, either by curettage or brush is preferred if the colposcopy is unsatisfactory or there are no visible colposcopic lesions.

Management of ASC-US in Special Populations

Management in adolescents (defined as young women aged 20 and under).

> The prevalence of HPV DNA positivity changes with age. Similar cytologic results will have different risk of CI2, 3 or cancer in different age-group of women

Adolescent women have high prevalence of HPV infection, more minor grade cytological abnormalities (ASC-US and LSIL) and are at low risk for invasive cancer compared to older women.[50]

The HPV infection in the adolescent has little long-term clinical significance, as majority of HPV infection clears spontaneously within 2 years after HPV infection. HPV testing to manage adolescents with ASC-US would refer large number of women at low risk for having cancer to colposcopy.

Therefore, HPV DNA testing and colposcopy are unacceptable for adolescents with ASC-US, as this can lead to unnecessary treatment. Even if HPV testing is inadvertently done, the result should not influence the management. In adolescents with ASC-US, follow-up with annual cytological testing is recommended. Referral to colposcopy is made only if persistence of ASC-US is reported at 24 months or HSIL or more is reported at 12 months.

Management of Postmenopausal Women

The 2001 guidelines recommended to use intravaginal estrogen therapy in postmenopausal women, who have ASC-US and to repeat the cervical cytology. Because of the lack of evidence to support this guideline, revised guidelines in 2006 recommended that postmenopausal women with ASC-US are managed in the same manner as women in the general population and use of estrogen therapy is removed. Only 20% of women aged 40 and older are found to be HPV positive. Therefore, triage of ASC-US using HPV testing should be proved effective.

Management of Pregnant Women

As the risk of cancer is relatively low among pregnant women with ASC-US, management of ASC-US in pregnant women older than 20 is similar to that of nonpregnant women. However, it is acceptable to defer Colposcopy until at least 6 weeks postpartum.

Management of Immunosuppressed Women

Recent studies have shown that the prevalence of CIN 2, 3 and HPV DNA positivity in HIV-infected and non-infected women are similar. Therefore, the 2006 guidelines recommended that HIV-infected and older immunosuppressed women with ASC-US are managed in the same manner as women in the general population.

Summary

1. ASC-US can be followed up with cytology/HPV testing/colposcopy in nonpregnant women aged 20 years or older.
2. Adolescents are followed up only with cytology. Colposcopy referral is made only with persistent ASC-US or presence of HSIL on follow-up.
3. Pregnant, postmenopausal and immunosuppressed women are managed in the same manner as women in general population.
4. Excisional procedures are unacceptable as an initial diagnostic procedure.

> For Indian population, limitations such as poor compliance, lost to follow-up and cost of HPV testing should be taken into account in deciding the mode of follow-up of women with ASC-US

Management of Women with ASC-H (Figure 11-2)

Studies have shown that CIN2, 3 lesions are seen in 40% to 50% of cases with ASC-H.[51]

Because of this high prevalence of CIN2, 3 in ASC-H, they are referred for colposcopic evaluation.

- If CIN2, 3 are confirmed on biopsy, they are managed as per consensus guidelines.
- If CIN2 or above is not identified, they are followed up with HPV DNA testing at 12 months, or cytologic testing at 6 and 12 months.
- If HPV DNA testing or 2 consecutive repeat cytologic tests are negative for CIN, they return to routine cytologic screening.
- If HPV DNA is positive or repeat cytology shows ASC-US or greater, further referral to colposcopy is made.

Management of Women with LSIL (Figure 11-3)

LSIL is associated with CIN2, 3 in 12%–18% of women.

In the management of LSIL, because of the high prevalence of HPV infection in this group of women, HPV triage is not useful. Also, because of the high incidence of CIN2,3 in these women, follow-up with cytology is insensitive. Therefore, colposcopy is recommended as the initial evaluation strategy except in special populations.

At the time of colposcopy, endocervical sampling is preferred in those cases in whom colposcopy was unsatisfactory, or colposcopy was satisfactory, but no lesion was identified. Endocervical sampling is also acceptable if the colposcopy is satisfactory and lesions were identified.

If CIN was identified at colposcopy, they are managed according to 2006 consensus guidelines.

- If colposcopy does not show CIN2, 3, either HPV testing at 12 months or cytologic testing at 6 and 12 months respectively is carried out.
- If they are negative, return to routine cytologic screening is recommended.
- If either the HPV DNA test is positive or if repeat cytology is ASC-US or greater, repeat colposcopy is recommended.
- Diagnostic excisional or ablative procedures are unacceptable in the initial management of LSIL.

Endocervical curettage (ECC) should be carried out irrespective of whether Colposcopy is satisfactory or not/whether lesion is identified or not.

However, ECC should not be carried out in pregnancy.

Management of Special Population with LSIL

Adolescents

Follow-up studies of adolescents with LSIL have shown a very high rates of regressions, nearly 90% in 3 years. Therefore, in adolescents with LSIL, follow-up with annual cytologic testing is recommended. Colposcopy reference is made, only if 12-month follow-up shows HSIL or more or 24-month follow-up shows ASC-US or greater. There is high prevalence of HPV DNA positivity in adolescents, which makes HPV testing of little value in this population. If HPV DNA testing is inadvertently performed, the result should not influence the management.

Postmenopausal Women

The prevalence of both HPV DNA positivity and CIN2, 3 declines with age in women with LSIL. This suggests that postmenopausal women can be managed less

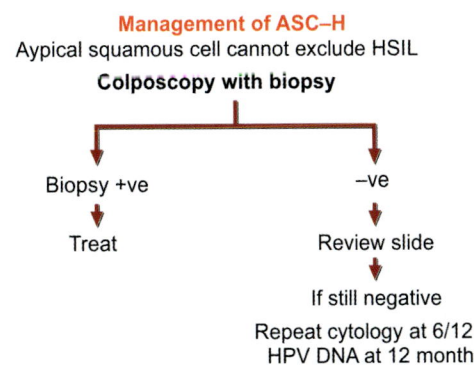

Figure 11-2: Flowchart showing management of ASC-H

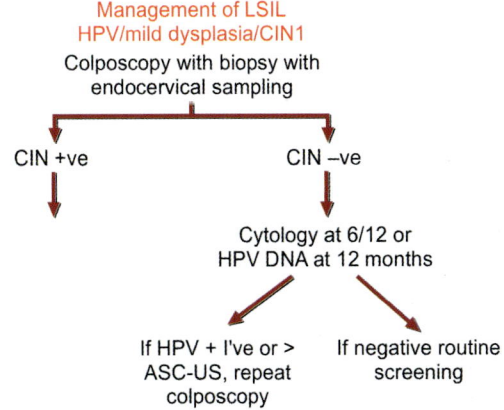

Figure 11-3: Flowchart showing management of LSIL

aggressively. The acceptable options for the management of postmenopausal women with LSIL include 'reflex' HPV DNA testing, repeat cytologic test at 6 and 12 months and colposcopy.

If HPV DNA is negative or CIN is not identified at colposcopy, repeat cytology at 12 months is recommended and return to normal screening with 2 consecutive negative smears. During follow-up, if either HPV DNA is positive or cytology is ASC-US or greater, colposcopy is recommended.

The use of estrogen cream to correct atrophy-related cellular changes is no more recommended. Instead, the use of HPV testing will allow differentiation between true precancerous lesions and atrophy-related changes.

Pregnant Women

In pregnant women with LSIL, colposcopy is preferred and the goal is to identify invasive cancer. The 2006 consensus guidelines suggested that the initial Colposcopy can be postponed until at least 6 weeks postpartum.

If colposcopy is undertaken during pregnancy, endocervical curettage should not be performed. When there is no cytologic, histologic or colposcopically suspected CIN2, 3 or cancer, they are further followed up 6 weeks postpartum.

Even if there is histological confirmation of CIN2, 3, pregnant women can be safely followed with colposcopy (to rule out invasion) until 6 weeks postpartum.

Summary

1. Women with LSIL are referred for colposcopy with endocervical assessment.
2. Adolescents with LSIL are followed up with cytology. HPV testing has no clinical use in adolescents.
3. In postmenopausal women, HPV triage/cytology/colposcopy can be used. Use of local estrogen cream is no longer suggested.
4. Pregnant women with LSIL are followed with colposcopy. However, colposcopy can be deferred until 6 weeks postpartum. If carried out, endocervical assessment is contraindicated.

Management of High-grade Squamous Intraepithelial Lesion (HSIL) (Figure 11-4)

The finding of an HSIL result on cytology is associated with 60% to 75% chance of having CIN2 or greater on biopsy.[52] Approximately, 2% of women with HSIL have invasive cancer.[53]

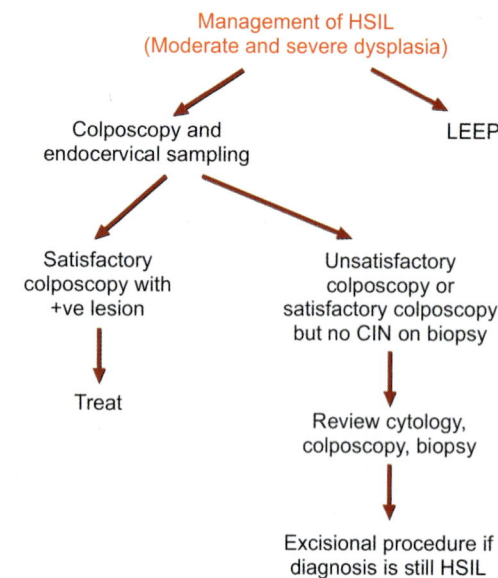

Figure 11-4: Flowchart showing management of HSIL

- As there is considerable risk of having CIN2 or greater is associated with HSIL, intermediate triage using HPV is testing or cytology is inappropriate.
- An immediate LEEP or colposcopy with endocervical assessment is an acceptable method of managing women with HSIL. However, many use see-and-treat approach using LEEP for initial evaluation. This method has been found to be time-saving and cost-effective for patients.
- In women who opted to have colposcopy, if the colposcopy is unsatisfactory, one should proceed with the excisional procedures.
- With satisfactory colposcopy, if CIN2, 3 is identified, they are treated as per guidelines.
- If colposcopy is satisfactory, but no lesion is identified, it does not necessarily mean that CIN2, 3 is not present. Therefore, one should review the cytological, histological and colposcopic findings. If the diagnosis is still HSIL, diagnostic excisional procedure should be carried out.

HSIL in Special Population

Adolescents

Adolescents with HSIL result should have a colposcopy.

As many CIN2, 3 lesions in adolescents and young adults regress spontaneously, LEEP procedure is unacceptable for initial evaluation.
- If CIN2, 3 are identified histologically, they are managed as per guidelines.
- When CIN2, 3 are not identified histologically, they are observed using colposcopy and cytology at 6 months' interval for 24 months.

If follow-up smear and colposcopy are normal on 2 consecutive occasions, they can return to routine cytological screening.

Excisional procedure in the adolescent with HSIL would be required only:
1. If the colposcopy is unsatisfactory
2. If the CIN of any grade lesion is identified on endocervical assessment
3. In case of colposcopically diagnosed high-grade lesion
4. If during the follow-up, HSIL persists for 24 months without identifiable CIN2, 3.

Management of Pregnant Women with HSIL

Colposcopy is recommended for pregnant women; however, endocervical curettage is unacceptable. Colposcopy should be carried out by clinicians experienced in the evaluation of colposcopic changes induced by pregnancy. Biopsy can be taken from lesions suspicious of CIN2, 3 or cancer.
- If CIN2, 3 is not diagnosed, re-evaluation with cytology and colposcopy is recommended 6 weeks postpartum.
- Even if CIN2, 3 is diagnosed, it is safe to wait until delivery, because pregnancy does not hasten the course of cervical dysplastic disease and the regression rate for CIN after delivery is high.
The route of delivery does not seem to influence the regression of cervical dysplasia.
- Diagnostic excision is unacceptable unless invasive cancer is suspected.

Management of Atypical Glandular Cells and Adenocarcinoma In Situ

Glandular abnormalities are reported as follows:
- Atypical glandular cells (endocervical, endometrial or not otherwise specified—NOS)
- Atypical glandular cells favor neoplasia
- Adenocarcinoma in situ (AIS)
- Adenocarcinoma

Atypical glandular cells can be associated with polyps, reactive changes as well as neoplasias, such as CIN2, 3, adenocarcinoma in situ, adenocarcinoma of the cervix, endometrium ovary and fallopian tube.[54] A study by Schnatz et al. has shown that glandular abnormalities were associated with high-grade squamous lesions in 11.1% of patients, adenocarcinoma in situ in 2.9% of patients and malignancy (Endometrial carcinoma, cervical adenocarcinoma and squamous cell carcinoma of cervix in 5.2% of cases).[55]

Because of the spectrum of Neoplasia linked to Atypical Glandular cells, evaluation must include colposcopy, endocervical evaluation and endometrial evaluation.

Initial Evaluation of Women with Atypical Glandular Cells (AGC)—NOS (Figure 11-5)

In the initial evaluation, colposcopy, directed biopsies and endocervical curettage are recommended. Endometrial sampling is also recommended in women older than 35, women of any age with abnormal uterine bleeding, women who are at risk of endometrial carcinoma (Polycystic ovarian disease, obesity). In recent years, HPV DNA testing has been included in the evaluation of glandular abnormalities.

The use of HPV DNA testing alone or a program of repeat cervical cytology is unacceptable for the initial evaluation.

However, the value of HPV DNA testing with AGC relates to subsequent evaluation.

If invasive disease is diagnosed during the initial evaluation, the patient is treated accordingly.

Subsequent Evaluation and Post- Colposcopy Management (Figure 11-6)

- Patients who have negative evaluation and are HPV DNA negative, they are followed up with repeat cytology and DNA test in 12 months.

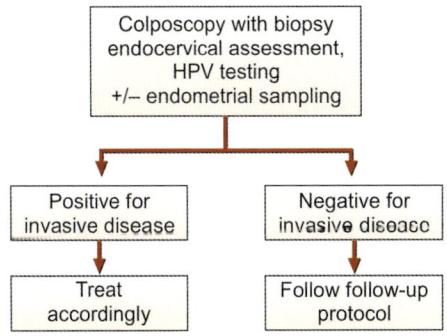

Figure 11-5: Management of atypical glandular cells (NOS) colposcopy with biopsy and endocervical assessment, HPV testing

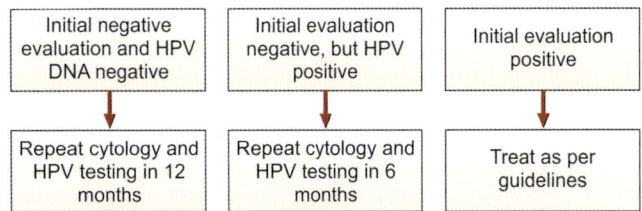

Figure 11-6: Subsequent evaluation and postcolposcopy management

- Out of those in whom initial evaluation was negative, but HPV DNA testing was positive, they are closely observed and repeat testing is done with cytology and HPV DNA testing in 6 months.
- If the previous HPV status is not known, cytology is repeated at 6 months' interval.

During Follow-up

- If both the tests are negative, return to routine screening
- If either cytology or HPV DNA testing is abnormal, complete evaluation is necessary.

Also Endometrial Sampling

- If endometrial cells are present
- Age > 35
- Abnormal uterine bleeding
- High risk for endometrial carcinoma (PCOD, obesity).

In those cases with a cytology report of atypical glandular cells, favor neoplasia or AIS, and if no significant lesion is found at the initial evaluation, excisional biopsy is necessary **(Figure 11-7)**.

The presence of endometrial cells in cytology smear in postmenopausal women should be investigated. An underlying hyperplasia or malignancy has been reported in 7% of the cases.[56]

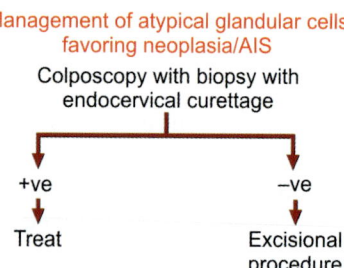

Figure 11-7: Flowchart showing management of atypical glandular cells favoring neoplasia

Evaluation of AGC in Pregnancy

Evaluation of AGC in the pregnant patient is similar to that of nonpregnant patient except that endocervical curettage is not done.

Only invasive disease needs treatment during pregnancy. AIS and CIN3 can be treated in the postpartum period.

Evaluation of Adolescents with AGC

Evaluation of adolescents with AGC is similar to that of older women.

Chapter 12

Colposcopy

An abnormal cervical cytology or positive VIA and VILI will alert the clinician as to the possibility of the presence of abnormal epithelium in the cervix, which can later develop into carcinoma.

The colposcope with its magnification and good illumination locates and defines the abnormality of the epithelium, stroma and its vessels. After locating the lesion, directed biopsies can be taken from these abnormal areas to confirm the diagnosis.

Following a screening test, if there is an abnormal Pap smear result or abnormal VIA or VILI, then colposcopy should be carried out as a diagnostic test.

Indications for Colposcopy

1. Abnormal Pap smear reports
2. Unexplained cervicovaginal discharge
3. Undiagnosed bleeding per vaginum
4. Lesion noted on cervix (even with negative cytology)
5. In utero exposure to DES
6. Persistent hyperkeratosis or parakeratosis in a woman who does not have prolapse or does not use pessary
7. Post-treatment surveillance of CIN lesions.

ABNORMAL SMEAR NECESSITATING REFERRAL FOR COLPOSCOPY

The presence of an abnormal smear should alert the physician that there may be a precancerous lesion in the cervical epithelium:

1. Any smear suggestive of invasive carcinoma
2. The presence of ASC-US (Bethesda classification) or mild dyskaryosis/borderline nuclear changes (BSCC) classification. Two such smears over a 6-month period
3. The presence of low-grade SIL (Bethesda classification)
4. The presence of high-grade SIL (Bethesda) moderate-to-severe dyskaryosis (BSCC)
5. Persistent unsatisfactory smears.
6. The presence of glandular lesion—severe glandular atypia/adenocarcinoma in situ.

CONTRAINDICATION

Any condition that would preclude vaginal speculum placement and inspection of the lower genital tract.

Advantages of Colposcopy

1. Identifies the source of abnormal cells in women presenting with abnormal smear; localizes the lesion for biopsy
2. Assesses the site and extent of lesion so that appropriate treatment can be offered.
3. Differentiates CIN from other conditions, such as infection which can give false-positive cervical smears
4. Evaluates subclinical papillomavirus infection (SPI)
5. Evaluates precancerous lesion in the vagina
6. Helps in the evaluation of abnormal smears in pregnancy
7. Helps in the follow-up women who have had treatment of CIN lesions.

COLPOSCOPY EQUIPMENT AND METHOD

1. Necessary equipment in the colposcopy room:
   a. Examination room that is adequate for performing colposcopy.
   b. Examination table (with adjustable height preferred) with stirrups.
   c. The table height should be comfortable for the examiner to maneuver the colposcope in front of the patient. Tilt-adjustable table is also preferred.
   d. A height-adjustable stool
   e. Mayo stand or table for surgical supplies
   f. Various sized Cusco's specula parous women would need wider and deeper specula; whereas post-menopausal women would require narrow and shorter specula. Very heavy and deep speculums will not stay and slip off.
   g. Autoclave equipment
   h. Gloves for the clinician and the assistant
   i. Solution for disinfection.
2. Equipment required for Papanicolaou smear
   a. Cervical sampling devices: Ayre's spatulas, cervical broom
   b. Cyto brushes
   c. Cotton swabs
   d. Glass slides and diamond pencils
   e. Fixative
   f. Transport container
   g. Laboratory form.
3. Equipment required for colposcopy procedure
   a. Colposcope
   b. Extra light bulbs for colposcope
   c. Lens paper to clean binocular lenses
   d. Ring or sponge forceps
   e. Endocervical specula (**Figure 12-1A**)
   f. Cervical biopsy forceps
   g. Endocervical curette
   h. Teaching head or TV monitor (optional)
   i. Camera for colposcopy (optional)
   j. Video attachments (optional)
   k. Specimen bottles
   l. Cotton-tipped applicators
   m. Roller gauze.
4. Chemicals and other supplies (**Figure 12-1B**)
   a. Lugol's iodine solution
   b. Monsel's paste
   c. Silver nitrate sticks
   d. 3–5% acetic acid
   e. Normal saline
   f. Cups for individual solutions

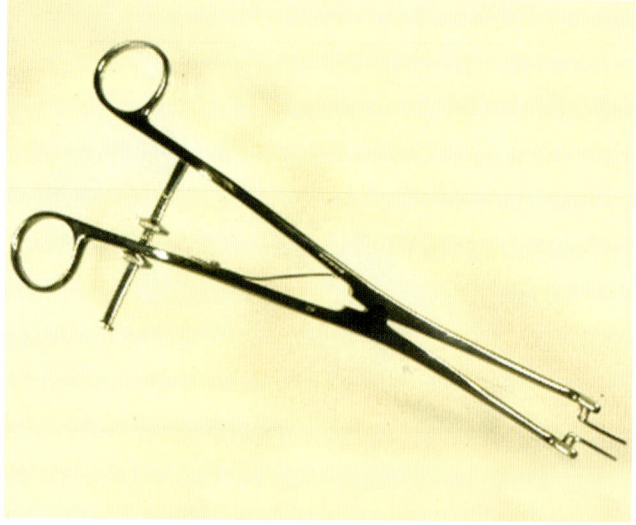

Figure 12-1A: Endocervical speculum

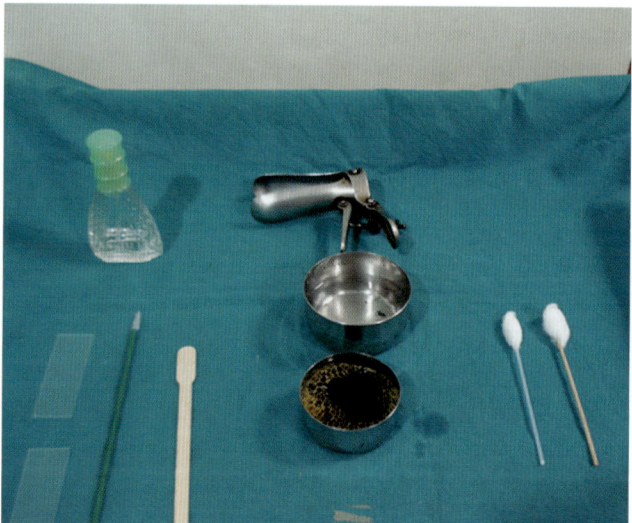

Figure 12-1B: Chemicals required for colposcopy

5. Required forms
   a. Patient information sheet
   b. Colposcopy form
   c. Clinical documentation and demographic forms
   d. Informed consent forms
   e. Laboratory forms for cytology and HPE.

THE COLPOSCOPY EQUIPMENT (FIGURE 12-2)

1. The colposcope is an instrument that provides magnification and illumination
2. It is a binocular microscope with a built-in light source and a converging objective

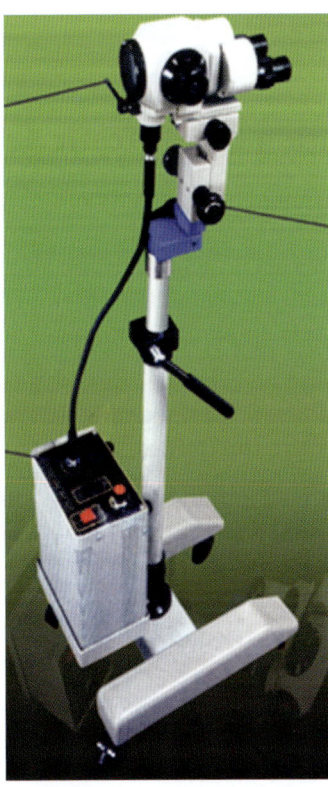

Figure 12-2: Colposcope

3. The lens:
   - The lens has a fixed focal distance
   - The focal distance is important because it determines the working distance between the lens and the patient
   - If the focal distance is too short, there will be limited room in front of the colposcope to maneuver the instruments
   - The lens with a focal length of 30 cms will allow examination of the cervix, vagina, vulva and anal region
   - The field of vision will be 30 mm to 40 mm.
4. The eye-piece:
   Two 10× to 20× eye-pieces are required
   Eye-pieces should be interchangeable
5. Zoom focus knobs:
   - Coarse focus can be achieved by moving the head of the colposcope closer or farther away from the patient
   - Zoom helps in continuous focusing throughout all the magnifications
   - Newer equipment have auto-focus facilities
6. Magnification:
   - Single magnification facility (4–12×) has limited capability for complete examination
   - Variable magnification has the advantage of scanning from low (5–6×) to medium (10–16×) to high (20× +) magnification

   a. Low power is used for the examination of the vulva
   b. Medium power is used to examine the vagina and cervix
   c. High power is used to detect fine vascular patterns
   d. If more than 30× magnification is required, the lens has to be changed.
   - The magnification will increase when the colposcope is moved closer to the patient, resulting in shorter focal length
   - Changing the magnification will change the diameter of the field of view
   - The higher the magnifications, the smaller is the surface area of the target tissue that can be visualized.
7. Green filter:
   - The colposcope is equipped with a green filter to enhance the vascular patterns
   - The green filter is usually incorporated into the colposcope head so that switching from white light to green filter is easily achieved
   - The green filter absorbs certain wavelength of light, making the red color of the vessels appear blacker and easier to see.
8. Light source:
   - The 15 V–24 V halogen light provides a brighter light
   - The light may be passed through a fiberoptic cable, which reduces the heat during the procedure.
   - Watts: 150 W to 300 W is used.
   - The illumination is adjustable with variable light intensities
   - The light source can be from single or double outlet.
9. Mounting the colposcope:
   - It can be mounted by a swivel arm on the wall or on a stand
   - If space is a constraint, a wall swivel mount may be preferable
   - Some clinicians do not prefer a stand directly in front of them
   - There will be tilting adjustment up to 50 degrees on all angles.
10. For teaching purposes, a beam splitter is incorporated between the binocular tube and the microscope body allowing for co-observation.

Digital Video Colposcopy (Figure 12-3)

- High resolution >850 lines
- Cold LED light source
- Digital Matrix Processor
- Electronic green filter with no light loss
- Timer
- >11.2 megapixels
- Magnification up to 42×

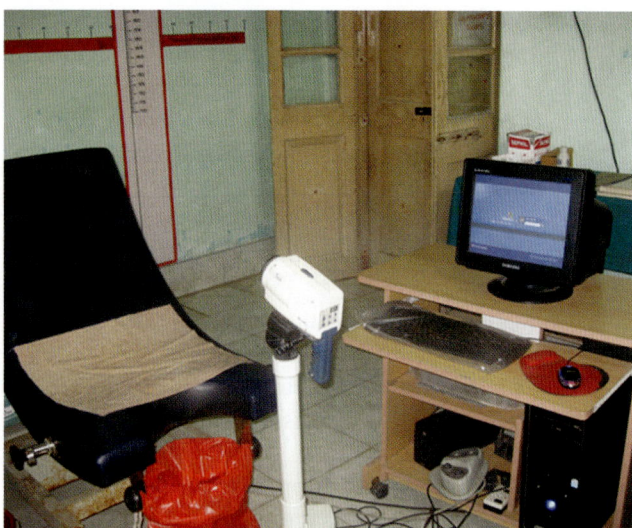

Figure 12-3: Video colposcope

- Real-time display of magnification
- Advance and auto-focusing technology
- Acetic acid test timer
- Image processing software
- The software is developed by the software professional with the following functions: view, image capture, image freeze, video recording, observation and processing. The pictures can be measured.
- Data can be stored as per the storage capacity of the computer.
- The pictures can be visualized on the computer screen, stored and recalled when required.
- One of the important advantages of the video colposcope is that you need not look into the colposcope and the field can be visualized on the screen and also can be seen by others and very useful for teaching purposes.

MAINTENANCE

- After use, always close the objective lens and eye-piece with the caps supplied and also fully cover the equipment with cloth—necessary to avoid dust deposit
- The lens should be wiped with spirit every alternate day.
- The colposcope should be wiped thoroughly every week.

1. CHEMICALS USED DURING COLPOSCOPY

1. Acetic acid or vinegar (3–5%)
2. Lugol's iodine solution
3. Monsel's solution
4. Silver nitrate sticks.

1. Preparation of 5% Acetic Acid

5% acetic acid should be prepared from glacial acetic acid, which is concentrated

- To prepare 5% acetic acid, add 5 mL of acetic acid into 95 mL of distilled water and mix thoroughly
- The solution is applied with sponges, large swabs or spray bottle.

Caution: **Undiluted glacial acetic acid causes severe chemical burns to the tissues**.

- It is left in contact with the tissue for at least one minute.
  Storage: Unused 5% acetic acid should be discarded at the end of the day.

2. Lugol's Iodine Solution

- Available in the market as Aqueous Lugol's solution and should be diluted to quarter to half strength (full strength solution causes irritation)
- Can also be prepared in the labs.

Ingredients

1. Potassium iodide : 10 g
2. Iodine crystals : 5 g
3. Distilled water : 100 mL

Preparation

A. Dissolve 10 g potassium iodide in 100 mL of distilled water
B. Add 5 g iodine crystals while shaking
C. Filter and store in an airtight brown bottle.

Storage

Lugol's solution is unstable and should be replaced every 3–6 months.

3. Monsel's Solution

- A ferric subsulfate solution which is used for hemostasis after biopsy
- Comes as a dark brown suspension
- Monsel's paste can be purchased (already dehydrated)
- If not available, Monsel's paste can be prepared in the laboratories.

Ingredients

1. Ferric sulfate base: 15 g
2. Ferrous sulfate powder
3. Sterile water: 10 mL
4. Glycerin starch: 12 g.

The Reaction May Emit Heat

a. Add a few grains of ferrous sulfate powder to 10 mL of sterile water and shake well
b. Dissolve ferric sulfate base in the solution and mix well
c. Slowly add ferric sulfate mixture to glycerol starch
d. Store in 25 mL brown glass bottle
e. For clinical use, allow the solution to evaporate until it becomes sticky in consistency which may take 2 to 3 weeks' time. At the time of use, very thick sterile water can be added to thin it.
    - The Monsel's paste will interfere with biopsy interpretation
    - Therefore, use Monsel's paste after all biopsies have been taken
    - The patient should be warned that the Monsel's solution may produce a charcoal vaginal discharge for the first several days
    - Storage: 6 months.

4. Silver Nitrate Sticks

- Used for hemostasis, but the patient may notice more irritation or burning than with the use of Monsel's paste.
- The silver will interfere with Biopsy interpretation.

2. EFFECT OF ACETIC ACID ON CERVICAL EPITHELIUM

3–5% acetic acid application:
- Before acetic acid application, the normal translucent epithelium reflects the underlying vascular connective tissue
- Squamous epithelium appears pale pink due to multiple layer of cells
- Columnar epithelium appears bright red due to single layer cell
- When acetic acid is applied, it coagulates the cellular protein, especially the cytokeratin, this biochemical change is seen through the colposcope as a whitening or opaqueness occurring within the visible epithelium **(Figure 12-4)**
- This change is transient and reversible
- Normal epithelium has minimal amount of protein and large amounts of glycogen.

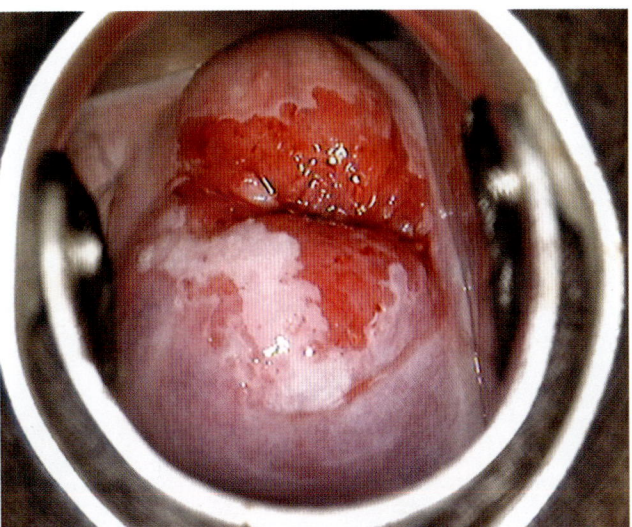

Figure 12-4: Acetowhite area on the posterior lip

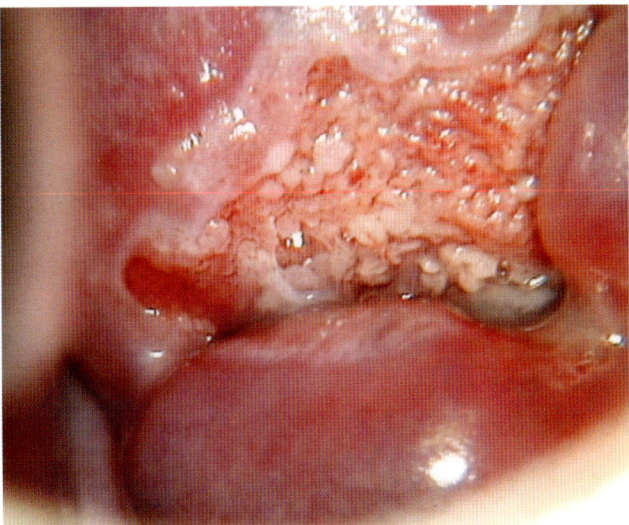

Figure 12-5: Faint acetowhite areas over the columnar epithelium

Therefore, when normal squamous epithelium is washed with acetic acid:
- It remains unchanged, retaining the translucent pink color
- The columnar epithelium because of the mucus content can become transiently white; however, the villi pattern will show the presence of columnar epithelium **(Figure 12-5)**
- In atypical epithelium, there is protein in the cell membrane, and increase in nuclear protein and very little glycogen. So, the squamous epithelium becomes progressively opaque and a dull appearance that masks the reflection of the underlying connective tissues will be evident. In major grade lesions the opacity of the lesion becomes more whiter **(Figure 12-6)**.

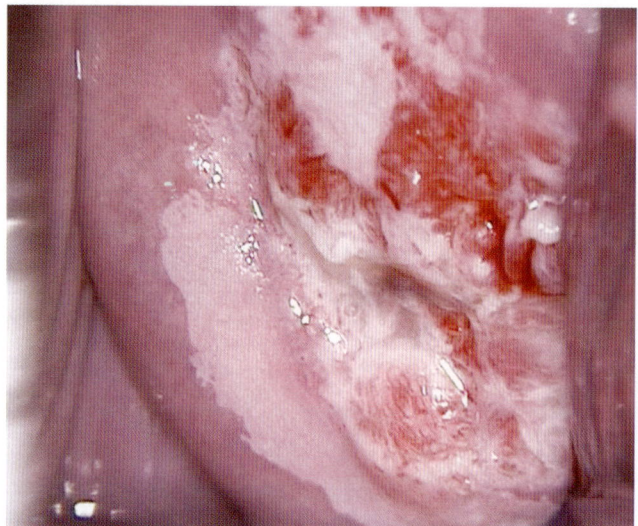

Figure 12-6: Dense acetowhite lesion on the cervix

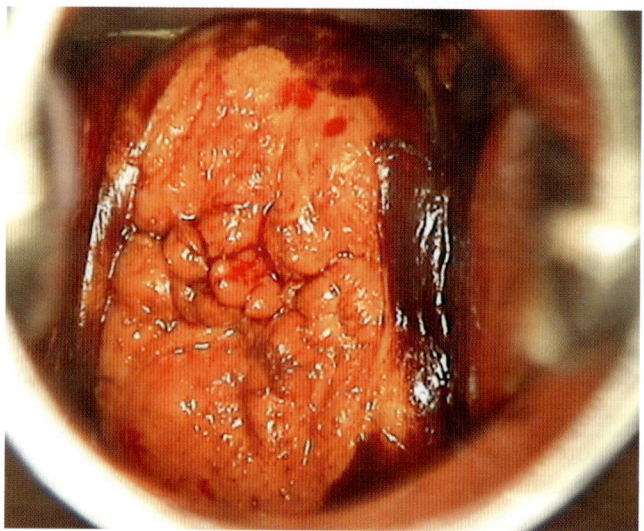

Figure 12-7: Wide iodine negative area

3. EFFECT OF LUGOL'S IODINE ON CERVICAL EPITHELIUM— SCHILLER'S TEST

- Normal tissues will have adequate glycogen content
- When iodine solution is applied to a normal tissue, a mahogany brown color appears
- Epithelium that contains little or no glycogen does not take up the stain (**Figure 12-7**) and will appear yellow.

PREOPERATIVE EVALUATION AND PREPARATION

The following history is taken from all women who undergo colposcopy, VIA and VILI

Name and address:

Demographic details:
Age, DOB and socioeconomic status

Menstrual history:
Menarche, menstrual pattern/Menopause in years and LMP

Marital history:
Married for how long, age at first intercourse, number of sexual partners, widowed, separated, remarried

Method of contraception:
Tubal ligation/IUCD/OC pills/condom/duration of use/when last used

Obstetric history:
Number of children, last child birth, age at first childbirth, MTP and miscarriages, last abortion

Past history:
STD in woman and her partner

Gynae history:
Periods regular/irregular/intermenstrual bleeding, postcoital bleeding abnormal vaginal discharge, previous gynae surgery, PID, itchiness/ulcer in the external genitalia

Previous cytology report

Previous treatment to cervix:
Biopsy, cryo, cautery

Social history:
Cigarette smoking or drug abuse

Medical history:
Immunosuppression—HIV/renal transplant/long-term corticosteroid use.
Allergies

Current medical problems:
Pregnancy test if there is possibility of inadequate contraceptive use

Evidence of infection:
Treat infection and then perform colposcopy
SE findings: Cervical polyp, ectopy, nabothian cyst, growth, condyloma, leukoplakia/contact bleeding at Pap smear

Postmenopausal women:
Use local estrogen cream for 7–10 days before colposcopy.

Informed Consent for Colposcopy

I, Mrs X, give my consent for the procedure of colposcopy. The healthcare personnel have explained to me the need for cervical cancer screening. I have been explained that colposcopy is used for the early detection of precancerous changes that occur in the neck of the womb (cervix).

The doctor/health-worker explained to me in detail about the procedure of colposcopy. I have been explained that the cervix will be examined under good lighting and magnification and the vagina will be washed with 5% acetic acid (vinegar)/iodine solution to look for abnormal changes in the cervix. I have been told that if there are abnormal changes, a sample of tissue will be taken from the cervix (biopsy) before the treatment is offered. Sometimes, the treatment may be offered at the same sittings, where the diseased portion may be removed by a minor surgery or destroyed by applying an ice-cold probe on the surface of the cervix.

I have also been told that the procedure does not require anesthesia, and the use of vinegar may cause some minimal irritation which is transient.

TECHNIQUE OF COLPOSCOPY

1. No anesthesia is required
2. The patient is asked to empty the bladder before the procedure
3. The patient is placed in the dorsal lithotomy position and draped
4. The colposcopist sits at the end of the examination table
5. The magnification and illumination are adjusted on the colposcope
6. The vulva and anal area are examined with the colposcope
   - Look for obvious condyloma or any other lesions
   - 5% acetic acid may be used to enhance the tissue
   - If abnormal areas are identified, biopsy is taken at the end of the examination
7. Cusco's speculum is inserted into the vagina
   - While inserting the speculumm, use saline as a lubricant
   - If indicated, take high vaginal swabs
   - Good visualization is an important part of colposcopic examination
   - In pregnant women and women with lax vaginal wall, the vaginal side walls may obstruct to view
   - To keep the vaginal side walls out of the field of view, use a vaginal retractor, or a condom may be placed over the speculum blades
   - Presence of mucus or active bleeding may interfere with the visualization of the cervix.
8. A Papanicolaou smear is obtained
   - If bleeding follows the cytological sampling, a cotton-tipped applicator gently placed into the endocervical canal will usually stop further bleeding
9. The cervix is soaked with normal saline and viewed with low power (4–10 ×)
   - Leukoplakia and gross lesions will be identified
10. Vascular pattern is examined with green filter
    - Acetic acid should not be used until the vascular pattern is looked for
    - Vessels are examined from low to high power
11. After ascertaining the vascular pattern, 3–5% acetic acid is applied to the cervix by spray bottle, through syringe nozzle or with cotton balls
    - Explain to the woman that it may sting a bit
    - Rubbing the cervix should be avoided
    - Place the cotton ball on the cervix and allow the acetic acid to thoroughly soak the tissue
    - The effect is transient and reversible
    - Repeated application is necessary as the effect peaks in 1–2 minutes and starts to wean off in 50–60 seconds
    - A second application of acetic acid, should follow the first to ensure a proper reaction
    - After applications of acetic acid mucus can be easily removed
    - Abnormal epithelium will turn white after the application of acetic acid (acetowhite reaction)
    - The acetowhite reaction will last only for a few minutes
    - As it fades, the vascular pattern such as mosaic and punctation will become more evident
    - Use high power to study abnormal vasculature
12. Now stain the cervix with 25–50% strength of Lugol's iodine solution and look for iodine positive and negative areas
13. Mentally map abnormal areas for future documentation
14. Endocervical Curettage (ECC): Wherever indicated, an endocervical curetteage is performed to evaluate the status of the endocervical canal
    - Under colposcopic guidance, curette is inserted into the endocervical canal
    - The entire canal is sampled rotating the curette to 360 degrees
    - Care must be taken not to contaminate the ECC with endometrial tissue
    - The curette should remain in the endocervical canal until the curettage is completed and the sample collected
    - Cytobrush may be used to remove the remaining samples from the OS
    - ECC should not be performed in pregnant women as it can evoke bleeding.
15. Ectocervical biopsy:
    - Biopsies are taken under colposcopic guidance
    - Benzocaine spray can be used on the surface of the cervix
    - The biopsy punch should be sharp
    - Make sure that lesion does not slip away as the biopsy is taken
    - Posterior lip of the cervix should be biopsied first to avoid dripping of blood obscuring the remaining biopsy sites.

16. Hemostasis following biopsy:
    - Apply Monsel's paste to the actual tissue rather than the blood oozing from the biopsy site
    - Apply Monsel's paste only after all biopsies have been taken. Histological samples become unreadable if applied prematurely
    - Silver nitrate sticks may also be used
    - Or after cleaning the vagina pack the vagina with roller gauze soaked in betadine ointment
    - Give strict instructions to the woman to remove the pack after 12 hours
    - Warn the patient that black discharge may be present for several days after colposcopic examination
17. Inspect the vagina as the speculum is removed
    - Look for any suspicious lesion and biopsy the area
18. If required, biopsy vulva and anal area
19. Bimanual pelvis examination is performed to assess uterus and adnexa
20. Colposcopic findings are documented as soon as possible
21. The patient is informed about the preliminary impression and given a date for follow-up.

Chapter 13

Interpretations of Colposcopy Findings

In order to interpret the colposcopic findings accurately, it is important to understand:
- The natural history of cervical epithelium, and
- The tissue basis of colposcopy.

NATURAL HISTORY OF CERVICAL EPITHELIUM

In utero, the fetal cervix has two types of epithelium:
1. The columnar epithelium derived from the Müllerian epithelium
2. Squamous epithelium originating from the vaginal plate epithelium.

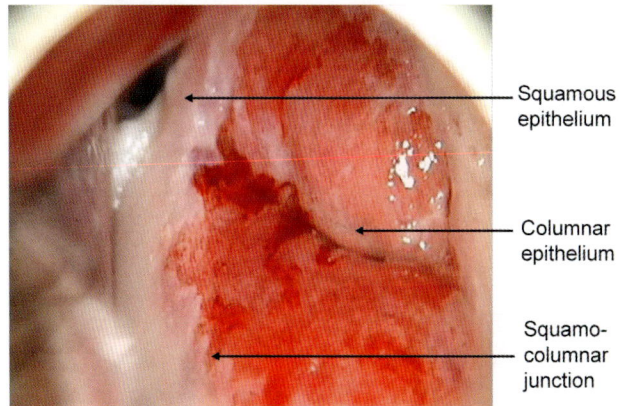

Figure 13-1: Squamocolumnar junction

I. Original Squamocolumnar Junction

1. The junction between the original squamous and original columnar epithelium is called original squamocolumnar junction (SCJ) and is at or just inside the cervical orifice **(Figure 13-1)**.
2. This original SCJ outlines the lateral (outer) border of the transformation zone.
3. It is fixed, but moves in relation to the whole cervix, e.g. as when eversion of the endocervical epithelium occurs in adolescence, pregnancy and injury to the cervix.
4. When the original SCJ moves outwards, the ectocervix is covered by columnar epithelium, which may sometimes extend onto the vaginal fornix.
5. When this exposed columnar epithelium is exposed to vaginal acidic PH, squamous metaplasia takes place **(Figure 13-2)**.

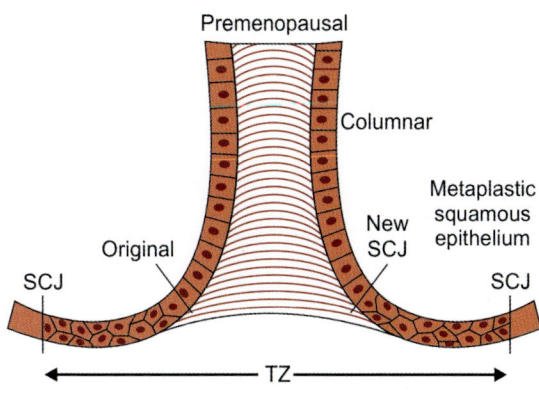

Figure 13-2: Squamous metaplasia

II. Squamous Metaplasia

- Squamous metaplasia is a normal physiological process by which columnar epithelium evolves into squamous epithelium.
- During the process of squamous metaplasia, initial event is immature squamous metaplasia, where there is marked proliferation of cells. This is followed by further maturation, resulting in mature metaplasia.
- During the metaplastic process, tongues of squamous epithelium may grow from the periphery into the columnar epithelium or squamous epithelium may surround islands of columnar epithelium (**Figures 13-3A and B**).

III. New Squamocolumnar Junction

- As a result, the columnar epithelium covering the ectocervix is now replaced by metaplastic squamous epithelium and this forms a new junction with the columnar epithelium of the endocervical canal.
- This is called the new squamocolumnar junction, and this outlines the medial (inner) border of the transformation zone.

IV. The Transformation Zone (TZ)

- TZ is an area of actively maturing epithelium between the original SCJ and the new SCJ. This zone shows squamous epithelium, columnar epithelium, and islands of columnar epithelium within the metaplastic squamous epithelium, gland openings and Nabothian cysts (**Figure 13-4**).

More than 90% of neoplasia occurs in the transformation zone. Therefore, colposcopic evaluation of the cervix will not be adequate unless the transformation zone is fully visualized.

TISSUE BASIS FOR COLPOSCOPY

The images seen through a colposcope depend on 3 morphological characteristics (**Figures 13-5A and B**).
1. Architecture of the epithelium, its thickness and formation
2. The composition of the underlying stroma
3. Surface contor

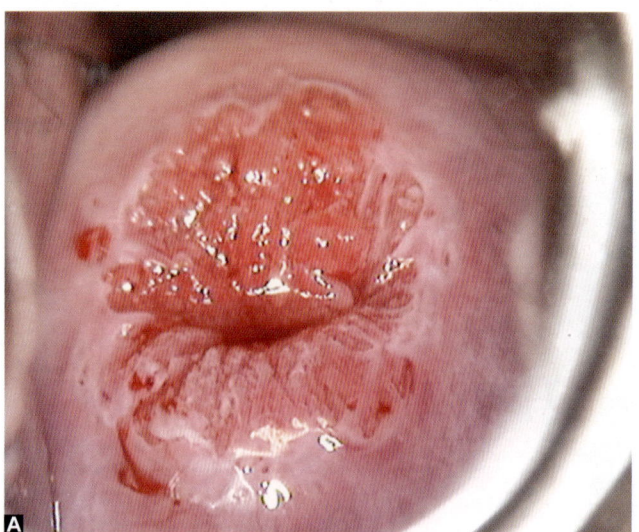

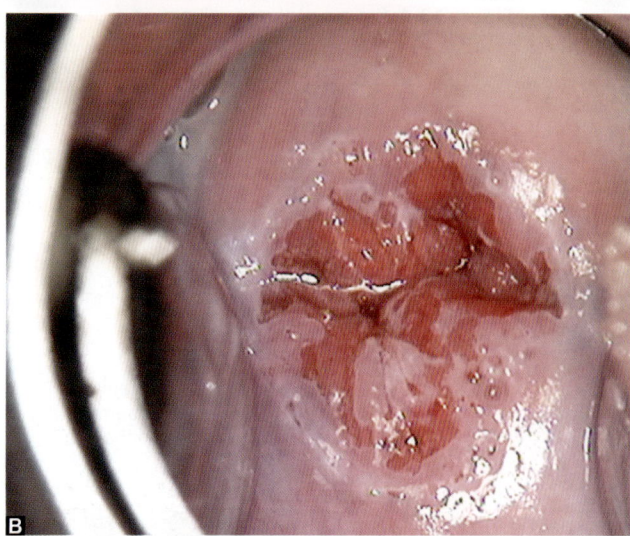

Figures 13-3A and B: A. Tongues of squamous metaplasia—squamous epithelium growing from the periphery into the columnar epithelium; B. Areas of metaplastic squamous epithelium within the columnar epithelium

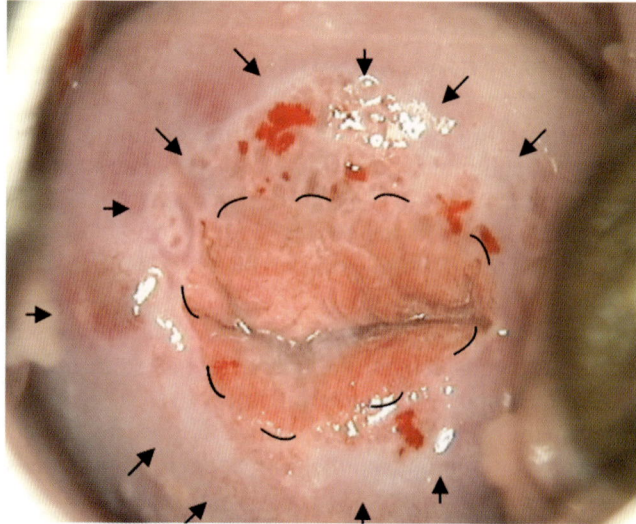

Figure 13-4: Transformation zone. Arrows showing the original SCJ and the interrupted line showing the new SCJ

Interpretations of Colposcopy Findings 53

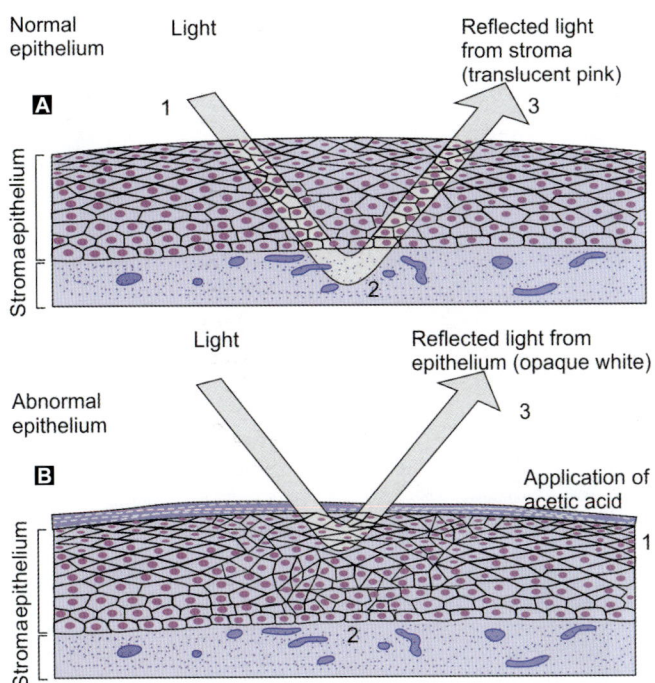

Figures 13-5A and B: Tissue basis for colposcopic images

The epithelium acts as a filter through which the light passes to produce the final colposcopic picture.

1. Epithelium

- The epithelium is colorless, whereas the stroma is colored by its underlying vessels
- When the light passes through a normal epithelium depending upon the thickness and architecture, the reflected light from the underlying stroma imparts a pink color to the normal epithelium
- Squamous epithelium
  During the reproductive years, the squamous epithelium is thick, multilayered and contains glycogen and acts as an effective filter; therefore, it has a pale pink appearance
- The columnar epithelium
  The columnar epithelium is thin, contains mucus, highly translucent and reflects the underlying vasculature in the stroma; therefore, it is bright red in appearance.
- Abnormal epithelium due to its thickness, increased nuclear content and altered architecture impart an opaque appearance after the application of acetic acid.

2. Stroma

- If there is infection, depending upon the degree of stromal inflammatory infiltration, there may be a yellowish or grayish white appearance.

- *Vessels:* Unless there are inflammatory changes or epithelium is abnormal, the underlying stromal vasculature will not be reflected on the surface except the color.

3. Surface Configuration

- Surface contor can be either smooth or papillary. Example: Columnar epithelium will give a grape-like villous appearance.
- Abnormal epithelium will have a nodular or heaped-up appearance.

INTERNATIONAL COLPOSCOPIC TERMINOLOGY

International Federation of Cervical Pathology and Colposcopy (IFCPC), 1990.

Colposcopic Appearance of Tissues

Normal Colposcopic Findings

- Original squamous epithelium
- Columnar epithelium
- Normal transformation zone.

Abnormal Colposcopic Findings (within the Transformation Zone)

Acetowhite epithelium*
- Flat
- Micropapillary or microconvoluted
  Punctation*
  Mosaic*
  Leukoplakia*
  Iodine negative
  Atypical vessels
  Colposcopically suspect invasive carcinoma.

Unsatisfactory Colposcopy

Squamocolumnar junction not visible
- Severe inflammation or severe atrophy
- Cervix not visible.

Miscellaneous Findings

Nonacetowhite micropapillary surface
- Exophytic condyloma
- Inflammation
- Atrophy
- Ulcer.

- Other indicated major or minor changes
  - *Minor changes:* Acetowhite epithelium, fine mosaic, fine punctation and thin leukoplakia
  - *Major changes:* Dense acetowhite epithelium, coarse mosaic, coarse punctation, thick leukoplakia, atypical vessels and erosion.

In order to accurately diagnose precancerous lesion of the cervix, the colposcopist must know:
- Whether the colposcopic examination is satisfactory or not
- How to recognize normal and abnormal colposcopic findings
- How to biopsy the abnormal lesion.

NORMAL COLPOSCOPIC FINDINGS (FIGURE 13-6)

1. Original squamous epithelium:
   This is clearly identified as a smooth pink epithelium without any features. There are no gland openings or Nabothian cysts. Stains brown with iodine.
2. Original columnar epithelium:
   Columnar epithelium is thin tall and single mucus producing cell layer. It is identified as an area with multiple villi or grape-like projections with a characteristic reddish color. Each villus has one or more capillary loops within a thin overlying epithelium. The red appearance is secondary to the proximity of the blood vessels.
   This tissue can be seen in endocervix or over ectocervix as erosion or in association with metaplastic epithelium. The pattern is best visualized after application of acetic acid. Columnar epithelium does not contain glycogen; therefore, does not take up iodine **(Figures 13-7A to C)**.
3. Transformation zone (TZ):
   TZ is the area of cervix and vagina that was initially covered by columnar epithelium and which by a process called metaplasia has been replaced by squamous epithelium.

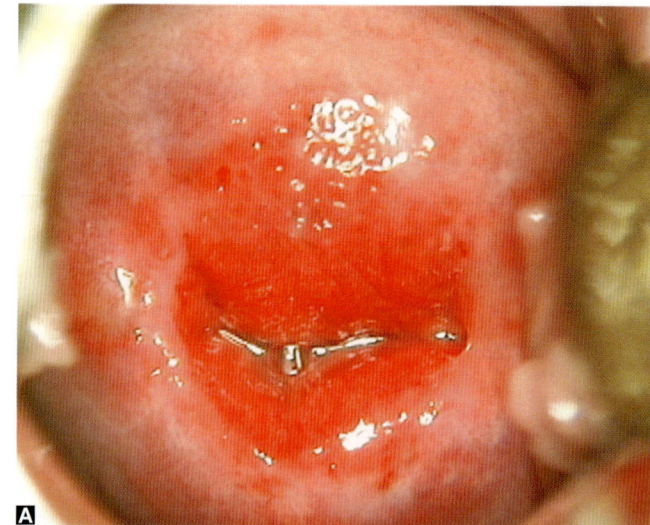
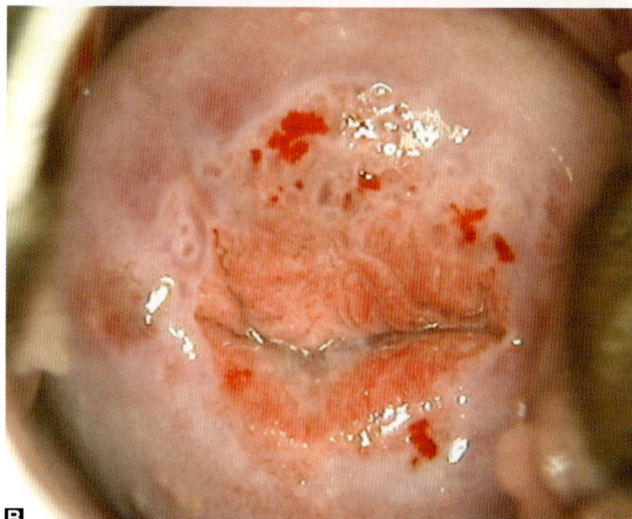
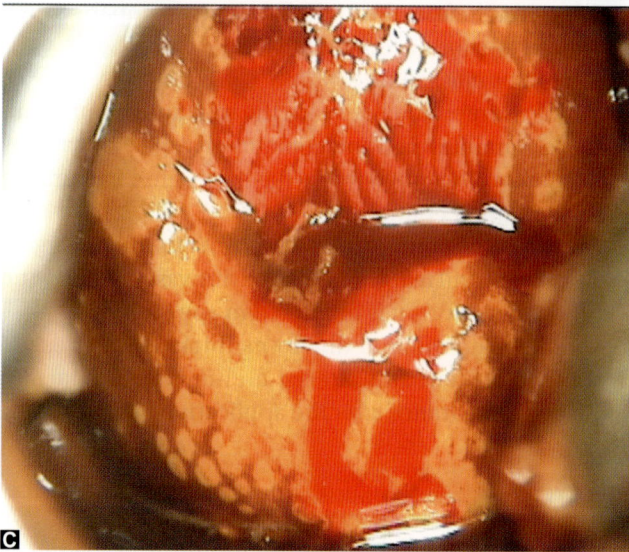

Figures 13-7A to C: Columnar epithelium on the ectocervix which is best visualized after acetic acid application. The columnar epithelium is iodine negative

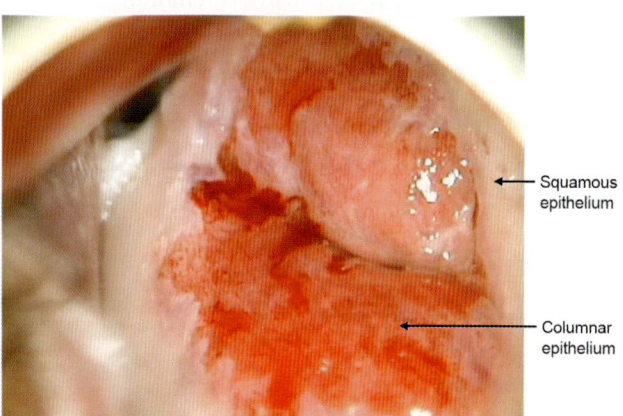

Figure 13-6: Squamous and columnar epithelium

This area lies between the original squamocolumnar junction and the new squamocolumnar junction **(Figure 13-8)**.

It contains gland openings, Nebothian cysts and Islands of columnar epithelium surrounded by metaplastic squamous epithelium **(Figure 13-9)**.

Within the TZ, squamous metaplastic epithelium may be seen from an immature epithelium containing 8–10 cells to a mature epithelium of 3–5 times thickness. In the stage of immature metaplasia, the cells are immature with intermediate and parabasal cells which have large nuclei.

After acetic acid application because of the increased nuclear protein content, it appears more whiter than the original squamous epithelium. The immature squamous epithelium also lacks sufficient glycogen; therefore, it does not stain with iodine. Because of these features, it is difficult to be differentiated from dysplastic epithelium.

In the stage of mature squamous metaplasia, it is difficult to differentiate between metaplastic and original squamous epithelium. However, presence of gland openings, Nabothian cysts and islands of red columnar epithelium surrounded by dense white area would indicate the metaplastic epithelium.

Vascular Pattern of Metaplastic Epithelium (Figures 13-10 and 13-11)

- Due to increased thickness, metaplastic epithelium does not reflect the underlying vasculature
- However, around the Nabothian cysts, the capillaries are often dilated, but have normal branching architecture. Sometimes fine network of branching vessels is seen.
4. Colposcopy of the adolescence:
   During adolescence, the cervix shows Typical TZ with original columnar epithelium and metaplastic squamous epithelium.
5. Cervical epithelium during pregnancy:
   During pregnancy, there can be eversion of the endocervical epithelium or gaping of the external cervical os, exposing the columnar epithelium to vaginal acidity and squamous metaplasia is activated. These changes are more likely to occur during the first pregnancy than during subsequent pregnancies.

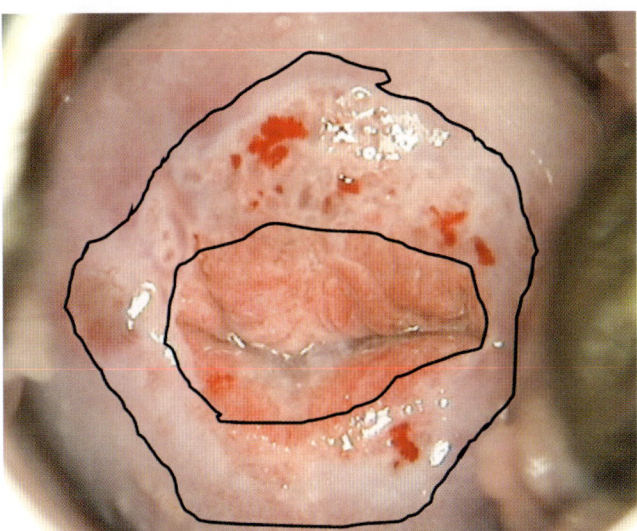

Figure 13-8: TZ between the original SCJ and new SCJ

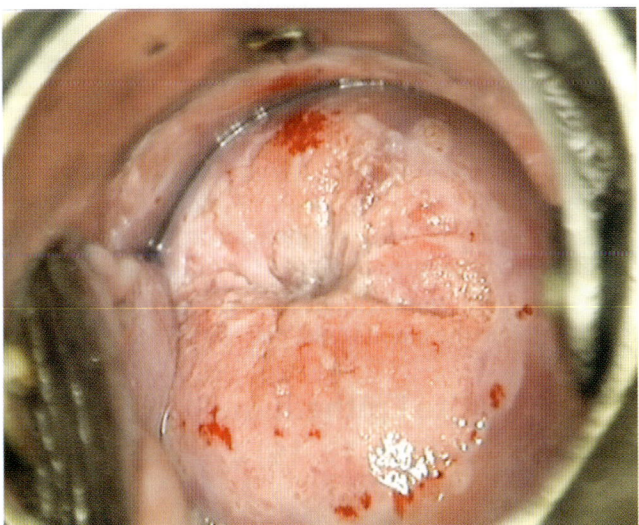

Figure 13-9: Metaplasia with faint acetowhite changes. An island of columnar epithelium surrounded by metaplastic epithelium is seen at 1 o'clock position

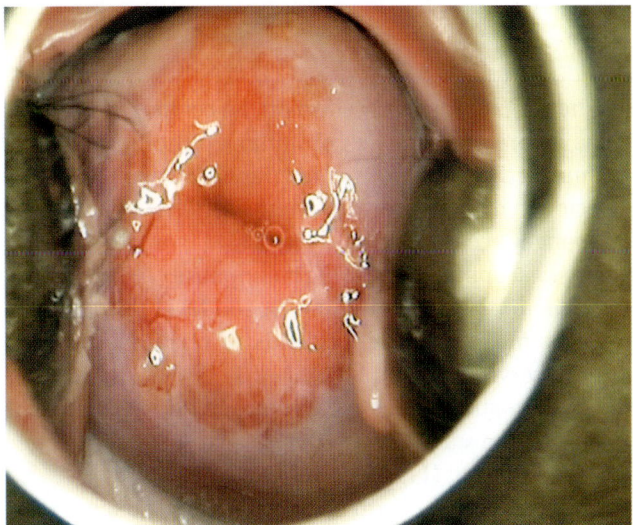

Figure 13-10: Branching vessels at 8 o'clock position in the metaplastic epithelium

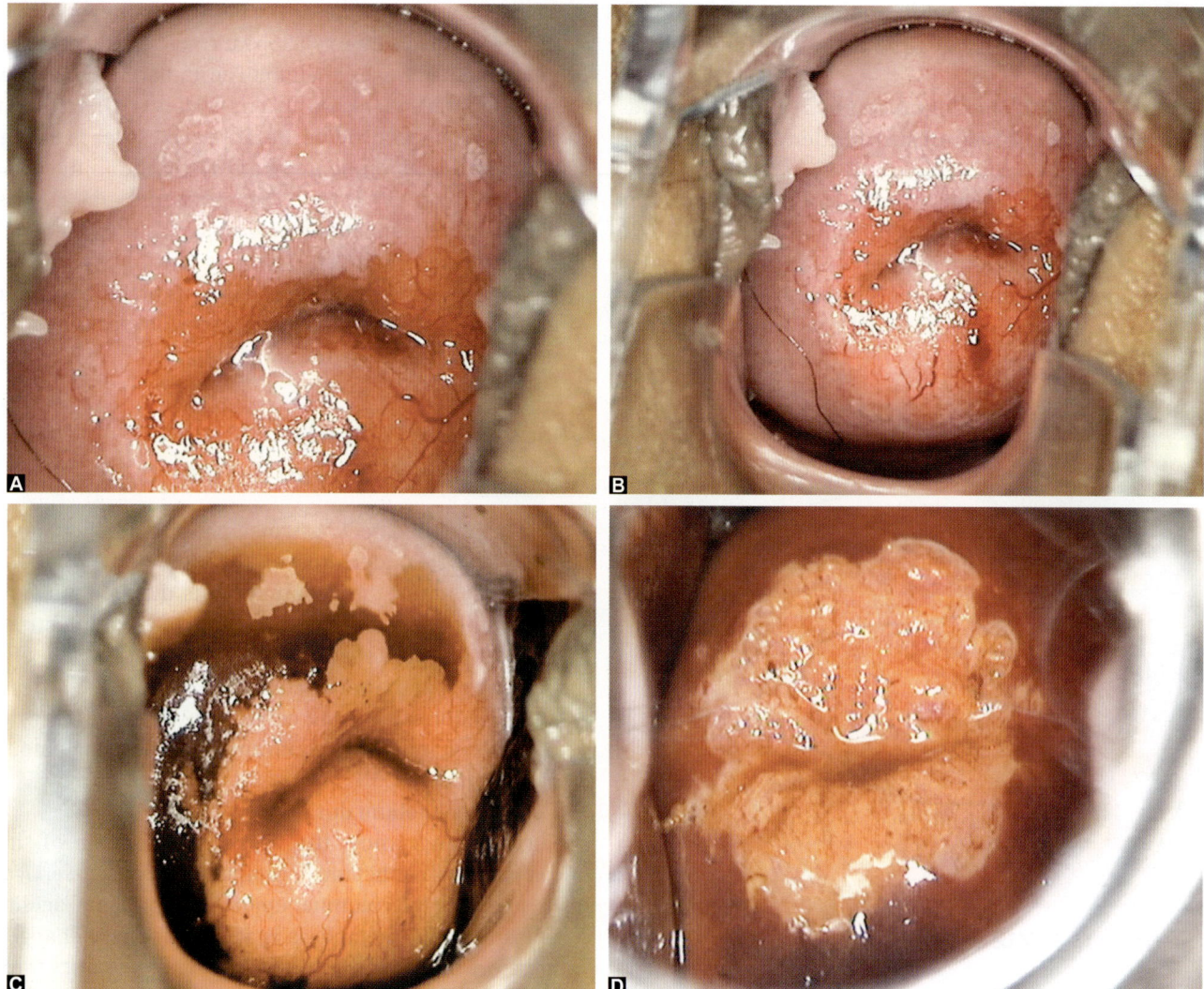

Figures 13-11A and D: A and B. Metaplastic epithelium shows faint acetowhite changes with satellite lesions between 11 o'clock to 1 o'clock positions; There is increased vascularity in the posterior lip. C and D. Metaplastic areas which are iodine negative

6. The OC pills and their effect on the cervix:
   As in pregnancy, the columnar epithelium and the supporting stroma are displaced outwards on the ectocervix causing ectopy or erosion where metaplastic changes occur.
7. Cervical epithelium during menopause:
   At menopause, when the estrogen level falls, atrophy takes place and the TZ tends to retract within the endocervix **(Figure 13-12)**.

   When atrophy occurs, glycogenation is lost and the epithelium stains light yellow and this loss of glycogen is not uniform **(Figures 13-13A and B)**.

   As the epithelium is atrophic, colposcopically underlying capillary network is easily visible and petechial hemorrhages may be seen **(Figure 13-14)**.

ABNORMAL COLPOSCOPIC FINDINGS

The colposcopic appearance of an atypical epithelium will depend upon:
1. The thickness of the epithelium and its nuclear content
2. Alteration in surface contour and any associated changes in the covering epithelium (Keratinization)
3. Variation in the blood vessel patterns.

1. Acetowhite Epithelium (Figures 13-15 to 13-19)

- Acetic acid causes the tissues, especially columnar and abnormal epithelium, to become edematous
- Acetic acid acts by dissolving mucus causing coagulation

Interpretations of Colposcopy Findings 57

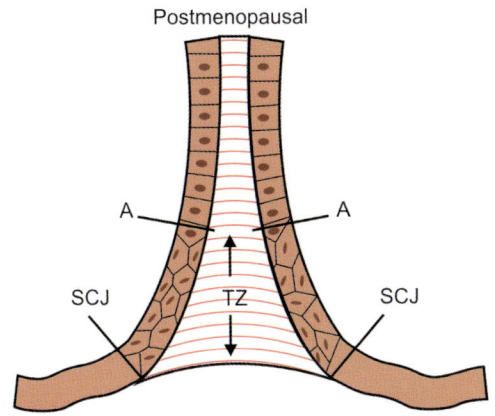

Figure 13-12: TZ within the endocervical canal in postmenopausal women

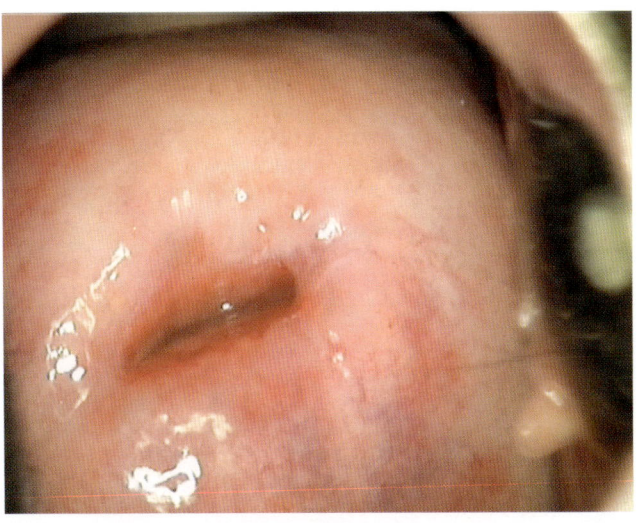

Figure 13-14: Postmenopausal cervix with the underlying capillary network

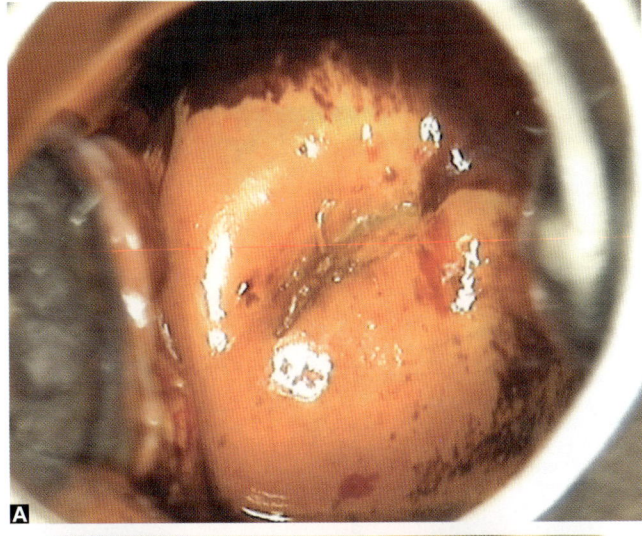

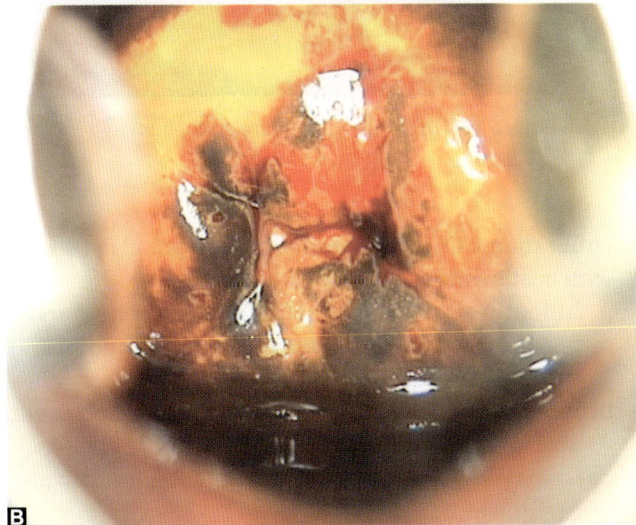

Figures 13-13A and B: Postmenopausal cervix with iodine negative areas

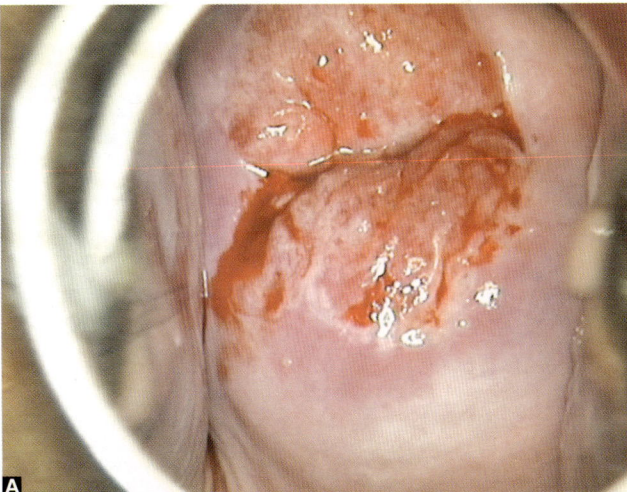

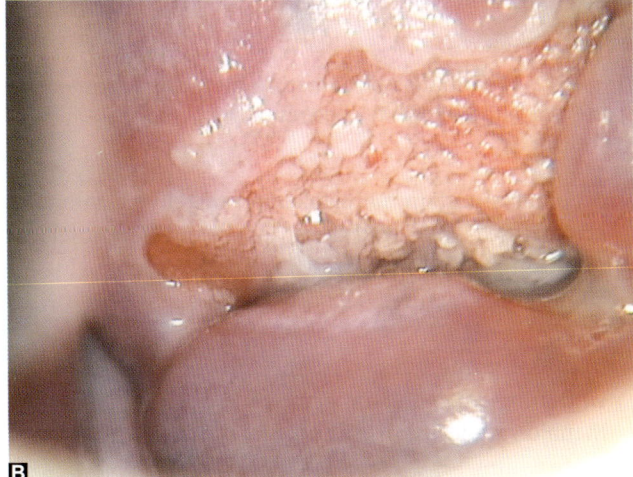

Figures 13-15A and B: Ectropion showing thin rim of faint acetowhite metaplastic epithelium at the periphery

58 A Practical Approach to Cervical Cancer Screening Techniques

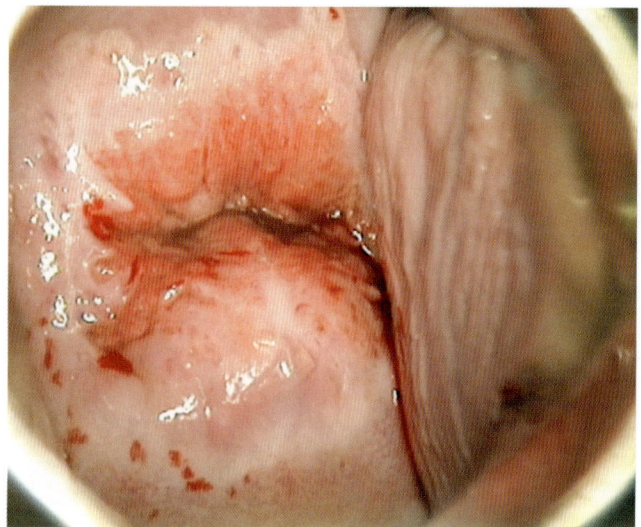

Figure 13-16: Pale, faint and translucent acetowhite changes of metaplasia

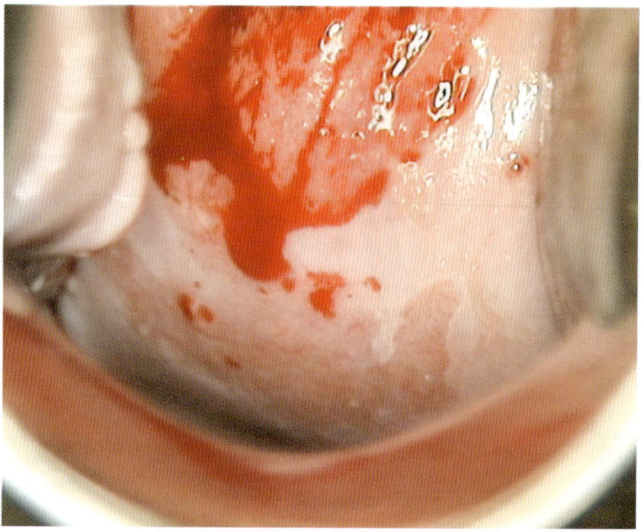

Figure 13-18: Thin acetowhite epithelium with geographical borders in a low-grade lesion

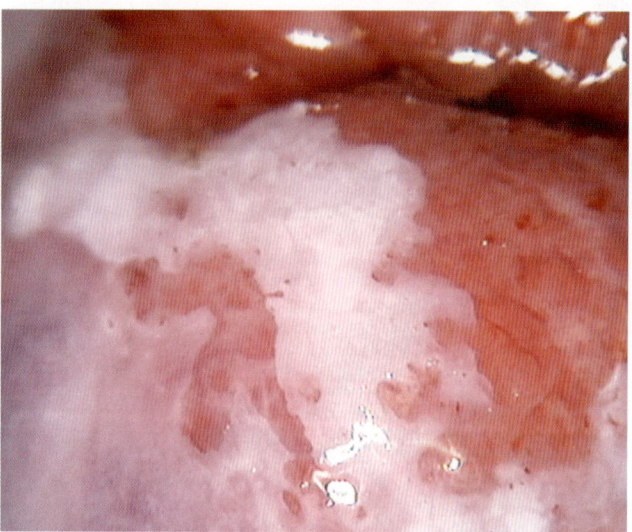

Figure 13-17: Tongues of immature metaplastic squamous epithelium with acetowhite changes growing into the columnar epithelium

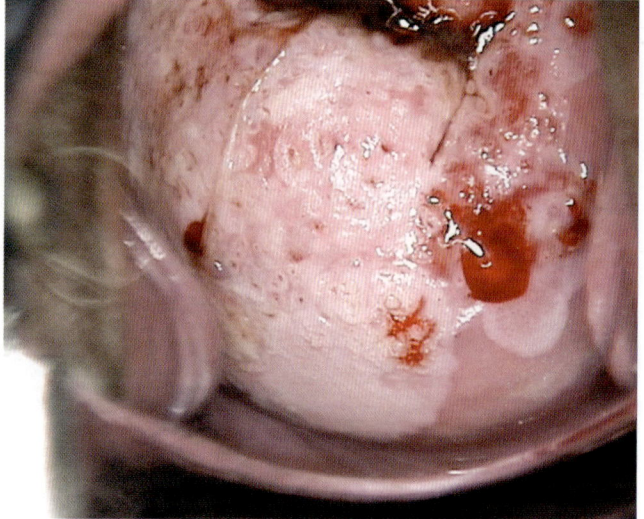

Figure 13-19: Dense acetowhite epithelium in a high-grade lesion

of epithelial and stromal cytokeratin, thereby accentuating atypical areas which will present as acetowhite epithelium
- Acetowhite changes are the most important of all colposcopic features because they are associated with all grades of CIN
- In minor-grade lesions, acetic acid will produce slight whitening and a dull appearance
- In major-grade lesions, the opacity of the lesion becomes more whiter
- A short while after acetic acid application, any atypical vascular pattern of punctation or mosaicism will become apparent
- Other than CIN lesions, other tissues can also present with acetowhite appearance:
  a. Immature squamous metaplasia—due to marked proliferation of cells and increase in the nuclear content of immature cells
  b. Virally induced lesions may appear white after acetic acid application
  c. Grape-like pattern of columnar epithelium will also become more evident.

So, it is important to differentiate these physiological and minor pathological changes from CIN lesions.

2. Abnormal Vascular Patterns

Abnormal vascular patterns seen through colposcopy are:
1. Punctation
2. Mosaic pattern
3. Atypical vessels.

1. Punctation (Figures 13-20 and 13-21)

- During the metaplastic process, the villi normally fuse. In abnormal tissues, instead of fusing, the villi remain separate and, around the individual capillaries, the abnormal nuclei proliferate, eventually compressing the villi, so that the tips appear as red dots.
- The vessels are dilated, often twisted and irregularly terminating vessels and are of a hairpin type.
- The area is usually well-defined so that a sharp line separates the normal from the abnormal epithelium.
- The punctation can be coarse or fine.
  This type of punctation is seen in:
1. Atypical epithelium
2. Also, when there is infection/inflammation, especially in relation to trichomonal infection and cervicitis. However, in these conditions, the dilated hairpin capillaries are usually diffuse across the ectocervix with no separate line between the normal and abnormal tissues.

2. Mosaic Pattern (Figures 13-22 to 13-25)

In the mosaic pattern, the villus pattern of the capillaries is lost and they are arranged parallel to the surface, interlinking with each other, forming a pavement-like appearance. The vascular fields enclose small to large areas of epithelial cells.

When acetic acid is applied, a pattern of white cobblestone is produced, each corresponding to an epithelial bud and surrounded by red margin representing the vessel.

When viewed from the surface, the wider the intercapillary distance, the coarser is the mosaic and the disease is more malignant.

3. Atypical Vessels (Figures 13-28 to 13-30)

Atypical vessels have a characteristic appearance and are associated with major pathological changes within the epithelium.
- Atypical vessels develop in the areas of punctation and mosaicism.
- The terminal vessels show irregularity in shape, course, density and caliber.
- Initially, the intercapillary distance within the precancerous tissue is reduced, but as the lesion becomes

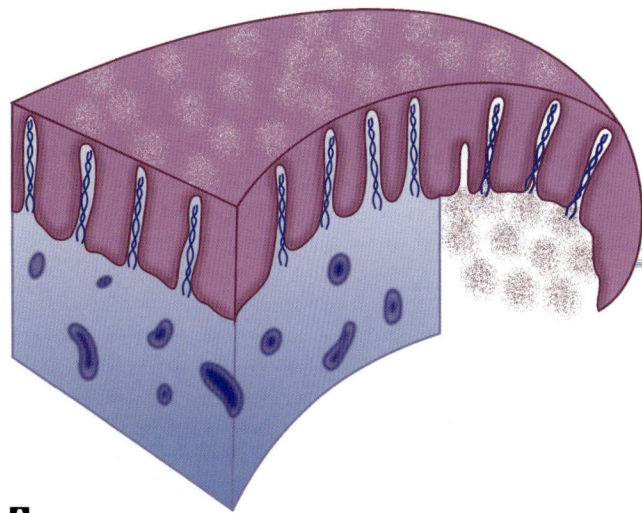

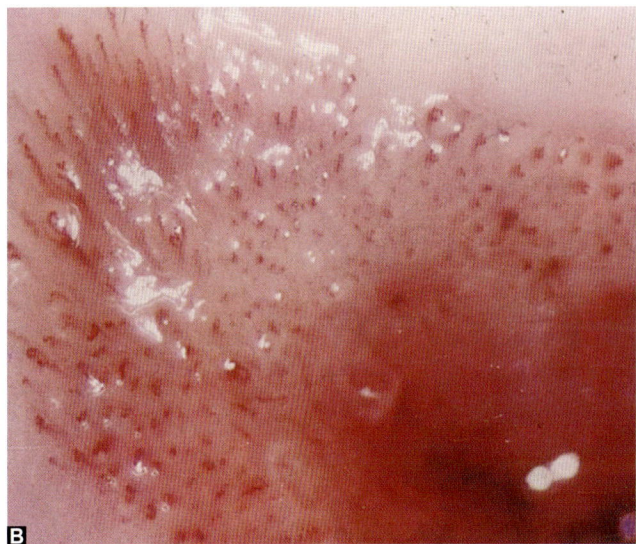

Figures 13-20A and B: Punctuation formation

more malignant, intercapillary distance increases and relatively larger avascular areas are formed.
- Atypical branching vessels never form the fine network seen in the branching vessels of the transformation zone.
- They do not have a regular tree-like pattern with reducing caliber as seen in physiological tissues.

Epithelial vascularity is best demonstrated using the technique of saline colposcopy viewed at 16× magnification, followed by green filter when the red blood vessels appear as dark objects and are readily visible.

Vascular patterns that could be seen in nonmalignant squamous epithelium are (**Figure 13-26**):
- Network
- Red-dotted
- Red-spotted

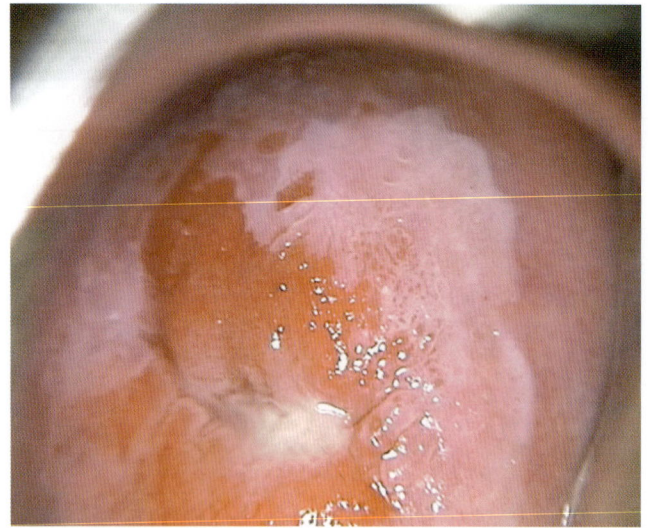

Figure 13-21: Coarse punctation at 2–3 o'clock position

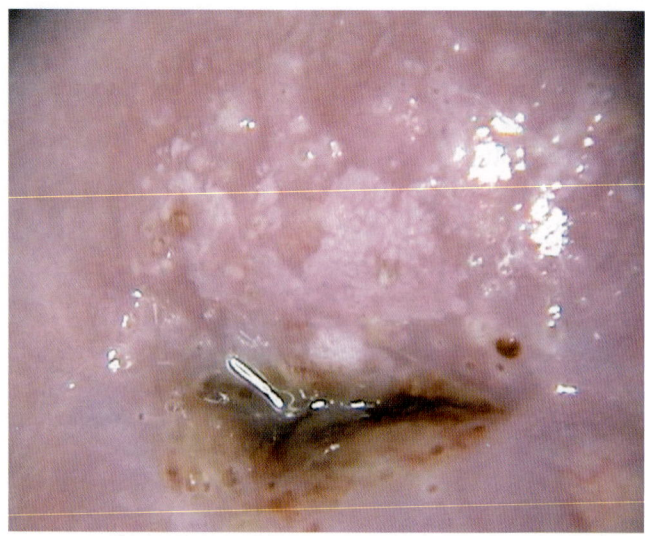

Figure 13-23: Coarse mosaics at 12 o'clock position

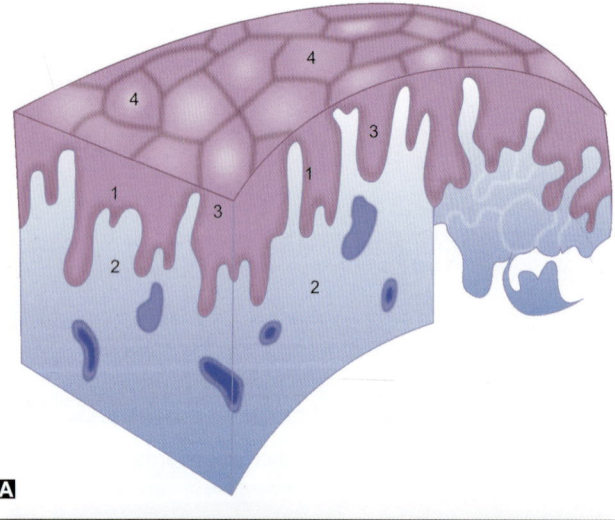

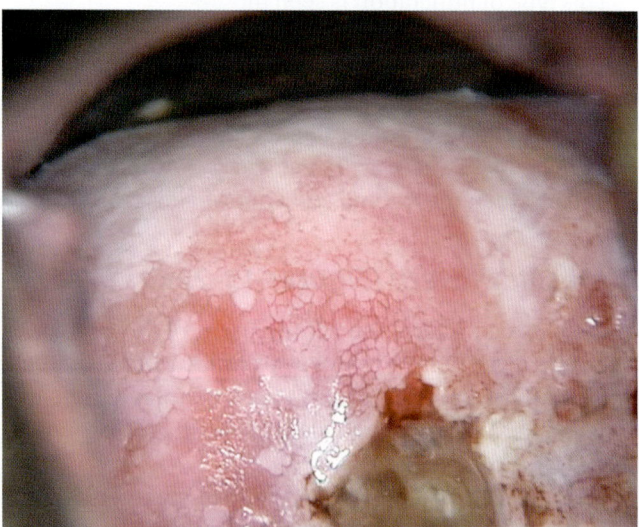

Figure 13-24: Coarse mosaics over the entire anterior lip of the cervix

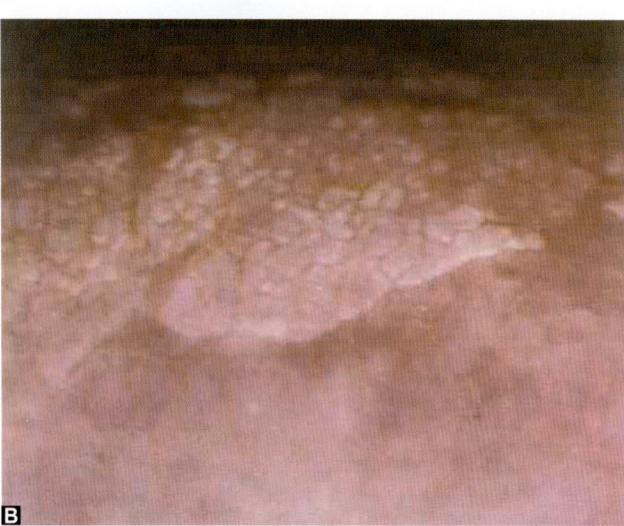

Figures 13-22A and B: Mosaic formation

- Branch-like
- Linear
- Loop like vessels.

In squamous premalignant and malignant lesions, the following vascular patterns are seen **(Figure 13-27)**:
- Glomeruloid
- Corkscrew-like
- Mosaic
- Tendril-like
- Waste thread
- Willow branch-like
- Root-like vessels.

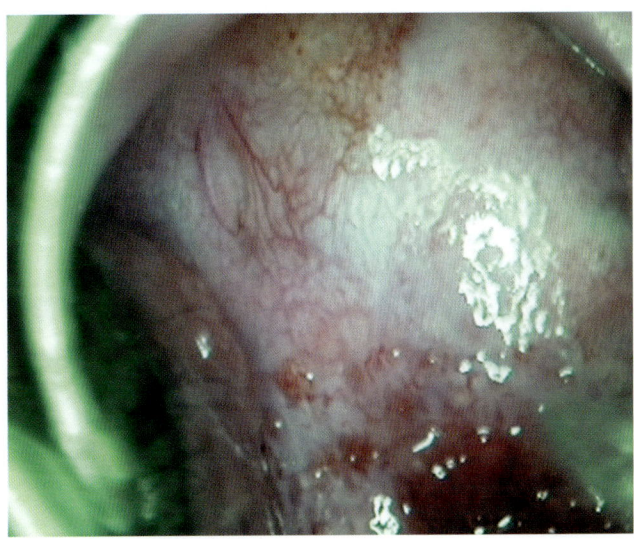

Figure 13-25: Appearance of mosaic through green filter

3. In Adenocarcinoma

Punctation and mosaic patterns are never seen
- Corkscrew vessels are seen
- Root-like vessels, tendril, willow branched vessels and thread-like vessels are seen.

4. Schiller's Test (Figures 13-31 to 13-33)

When iodine solution is applied to normal tissue, a brownish stain develops due to the inherent glycogen content. Epithelium that contains little or no glycogen content does not take up the stain.
- Immature metaplastic epithelium, atrophic epithelium and glandular epithelium, such as columnar epithelium do not stain with iodine as they are devoid of glycogen.
- Subclinical papillomavirus infection and abnormal epithelium, such as CIN lesions are glycogen-free; therefore, cervix stains yellow.
- After menopause, cervix stains light brown or yellow.

Other Features of Abnormal Epithelium

During colposcopic examination, one should also be looking for other features such as:
- Leukoplakia
- Surface contour
- Line of demarcation between normal and abnormal epithelium
- Location of lesion.

5. Leukoplakia (Figure 13-34)

- Due to hyperkeratosis and parakeratosis
- Typically an elevated white plaque seen prior to the application of acetic acid.
- Seen in conditions with chronic irritation, such as with prolapse uterus, pessary use or infection, such as HPV infection.
- Long-standing persistent leukoplakia should be investigated for underlying malignancy.

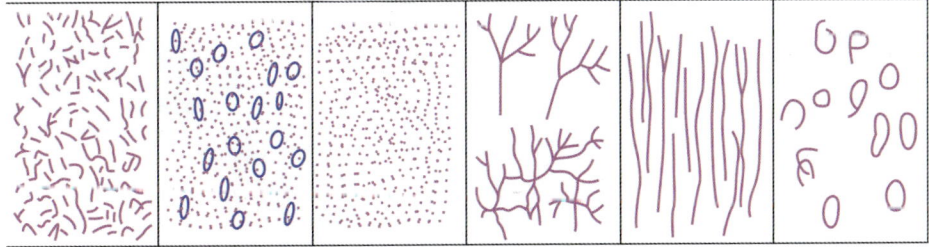

Figure 13-26: Vascular patterns in benign conditions

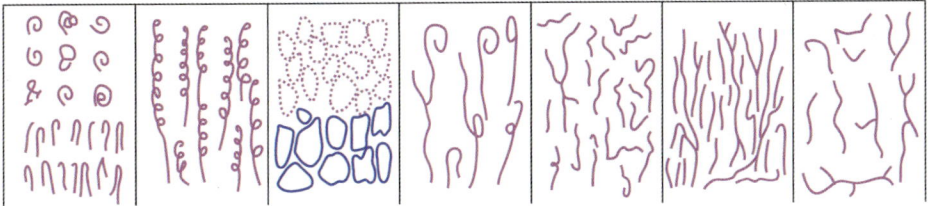

Figure 13-27: Vascular patterns in premalignant and malignant lesions of the cervix

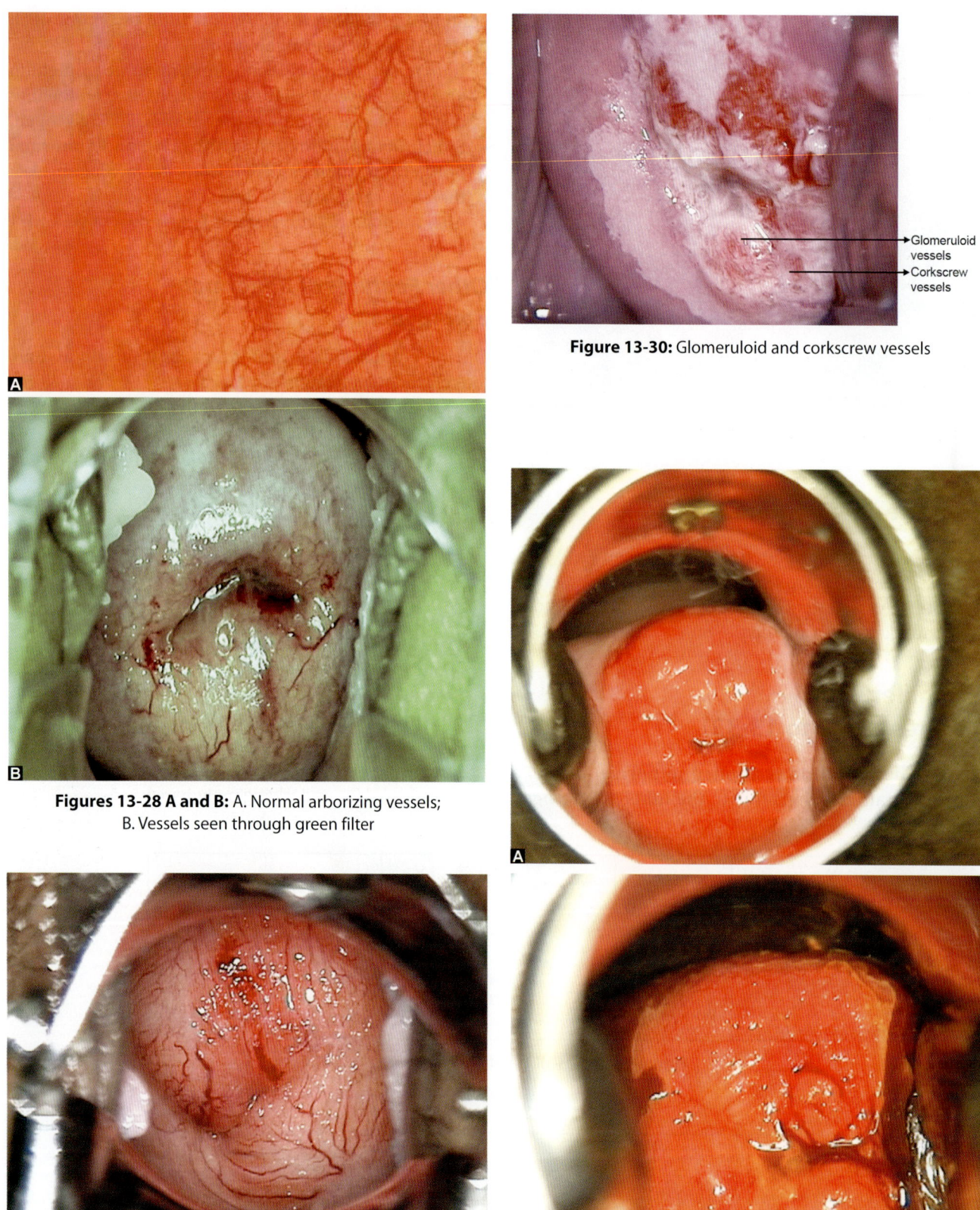

Figures 13-28 A and B: A. Normal arborizing vessels; B. Vessels seen through green filter

Figure 13-29: Parallel running wide caliber vessels in the cervix

Figure 13-30: Glomeruloid and corkscrew vessels

Figures 13-31A and B: Large ectropion and the exposed columnar epithelium is iodine negative

Interpretations of Colposcopy Findings

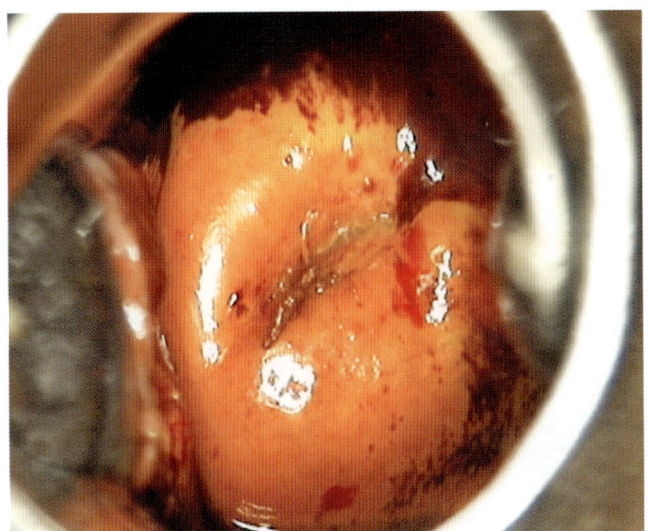

Figure 13-32: Iodine negative area in postmenopausal cervix

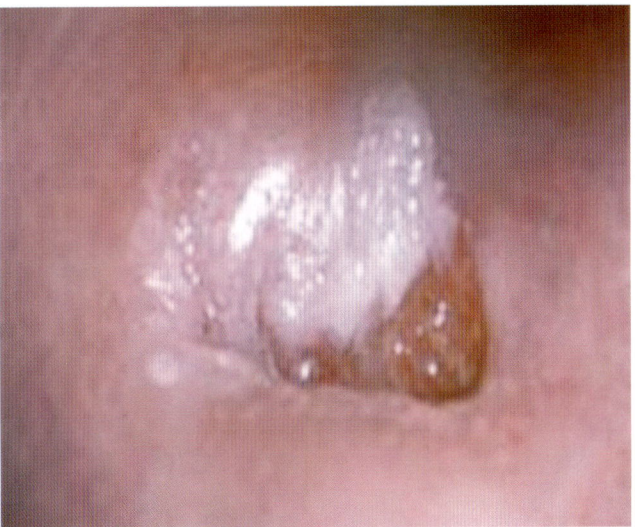

Figure 13-34: Leukoplakia

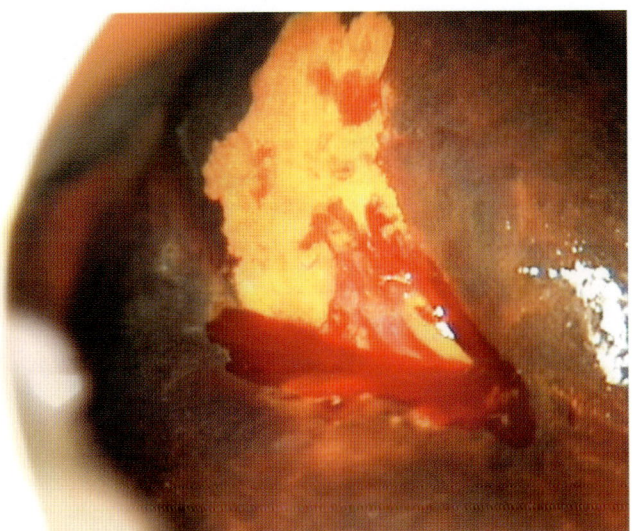

Figure 13-33: Well-demarcated iodine negative area in a low-grade lesion

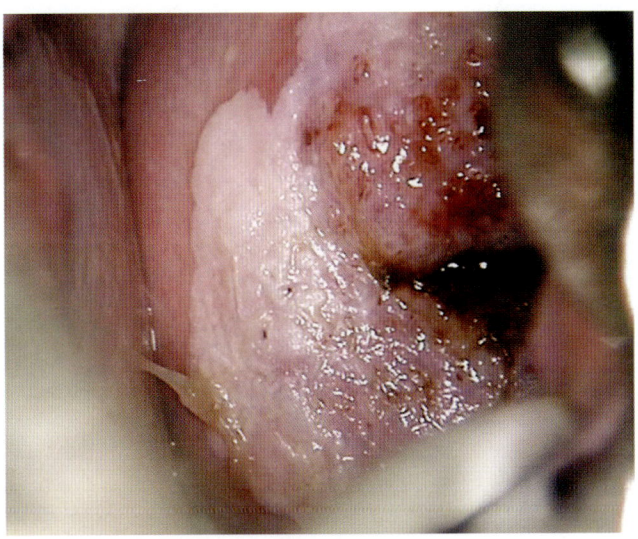

Figure 13-35: Elevated acetowhite epithelium in a high-grade lesion

6. Surface Contour

- Described as smooth, uneven, papillary or nodular
- Native squamous epithelium has smooth surface
- Columnar epithelium is papillary
- High-grade lesions are elevated (Figure 13-35)
- Frankly invasive lesions have a nodular or polypoidal surface that finally develop into ulcerated or exophytic growth.

7. Line of Demarcation

- The boundary between the native squamous epithelium and inflammatory lesions and lesser grades of CIN lesions are diffuse (Figure 13-36).
- Clear line of demarcation exists between the native squamous epithelium and high-grade CIN lesions **(Figures 13-37 and 13-38)**.

8. Location of Lesion

Lesions away from the SCJ and satellite lesions are most likely benign and HPV-induced lesions (Figure 13-39).

Abnormal lesions are close to the SCJ (Figure 13-40).

64 A Practical Approach to Cervical Cancer Screening Techniques

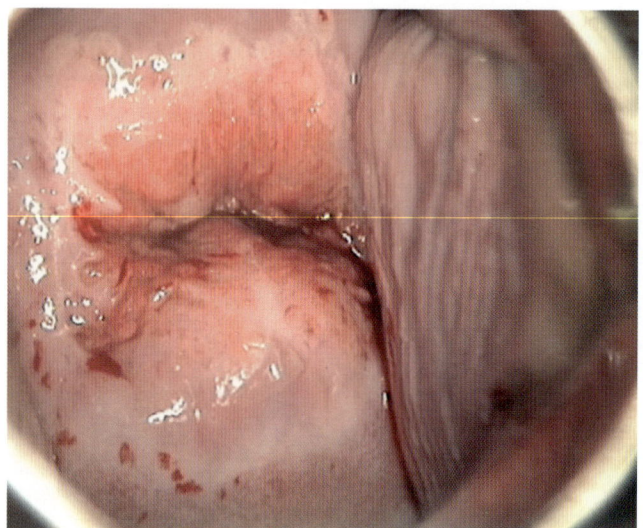

Figure 13-36: Diffuse, indistinct margins in metaplastic epithelium

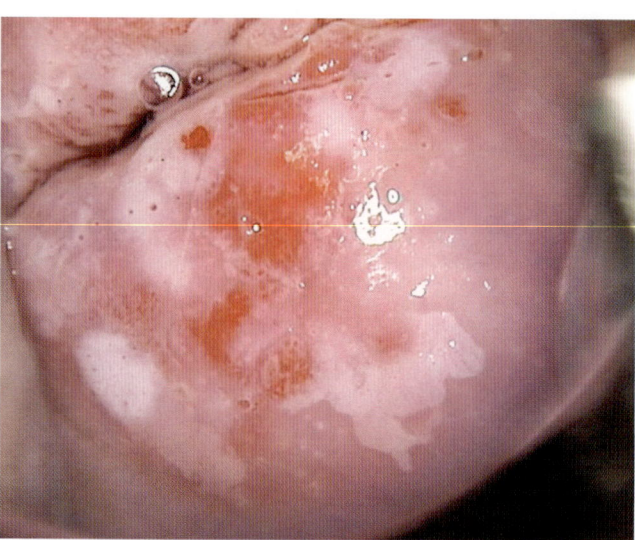

Figure 13-38: Indistinct margins as well as clear demarcation

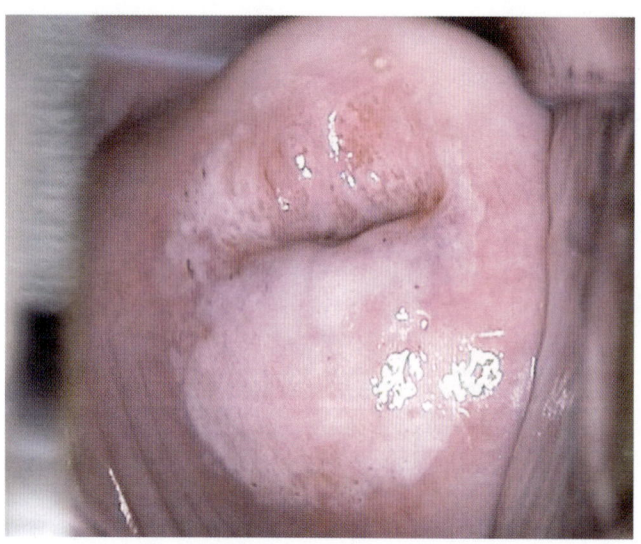

Figure 13-37: Clear demarcation between normal and abnormal epithelia

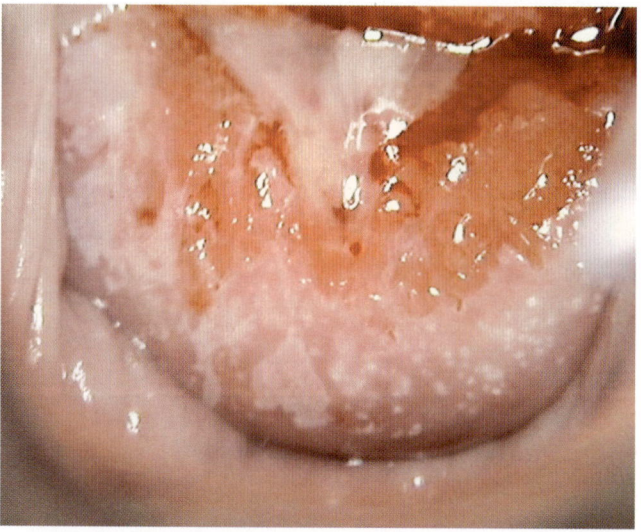

Figure 13-39: Irregular, angular, faint acetowhite areas with HPV- induced satellite lesions

SIGNIFICANCE OF ABNORMAL COLPOSCOPIC FINDINGS IN NON-NEOPLASTIC LESIONS

Abnormal findings such as acetowhite epithelium, punctation and iodine-negative areas may be seen in non-neoplastic conditions, such as metaplasia, infection, inflammation, regeneration and repair following trauma, cautery and cryosurgery.

Therefore, Pap smear and colposcopy should not be done within 3 months of injury or treatment to the cervix.

> The presence of atypical epithelium is highly suggestive but not diagnostic of neoplasia, therefore, confirmatory biopsy should be taken

Indications for Endocervical Assessment

- Either endocervical brush or curette can be used
- When the colposcopic examination is unsatisfactory
- When there is uncertainty as to the existence of

Interpretations of Colposcopy Findings

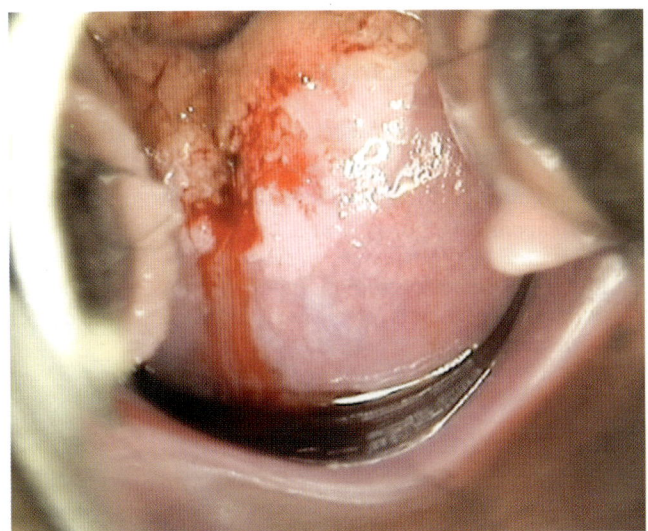

Figure 13-40: Abnormal acetowhite area close to the SCJ

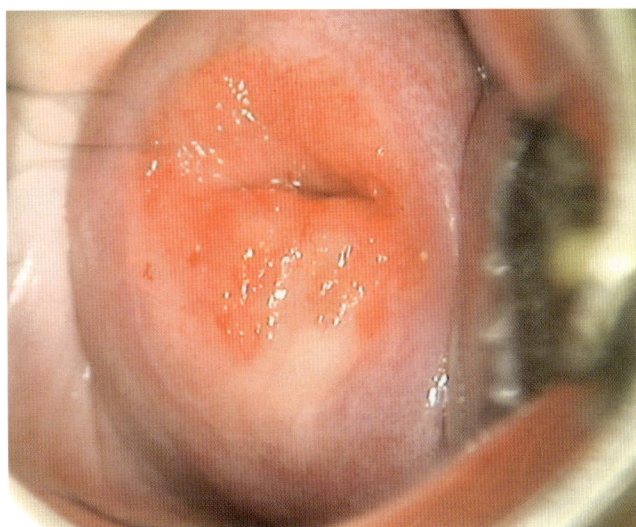

Figure 13-41: Satisfactory colposcopy—new SCJ is fully visible

unsuspected abnormality within the endocervical canal, above the new squamocolumnar junction
- After treatment of CIN—when the cervical canal is partly stenosed and difficult to see the new SCJ.

Disadvantages

- Circumferential scraping is necessary, so it is painful.
- Difficult to judge the relationship between the stroma and the epithelium
- No indication as to the depth of involvement of neoplastic tissue.

Contraindication

- Endocervical assessment should not be undertaken in pregnancy.

As the false-negative rates are high with endocervical curettage and brush, the endocervical sampling should not influence the management when the colposcopy is unsatisfactory

Satisfactory and Unsatisfactory Colposcopy

The most important part of the examination is to obtain:
1. Full topography of the lesion, identifying the outer and inner limits of the abnormal area
2. Morphology—precise identification and interpretation of abnormal colposcopy features.

Satisfactory Colposcopy (Figure 13-41)

When the new squamocolumnar junction and full extent of the abnormal epithelium are fully visible, then the colposcopic examination is satisfactory. Assessment of the inner limit is the most important part of examination.

Unsatisfactory Colposcopy (Figures 13-42 and 13-43)

An unsatisfactory examination is the one in which the new squamocolumnar junction is not visible/or severe inflammation or severe atrophy make it impossible to determine the inner limit of the lesion.

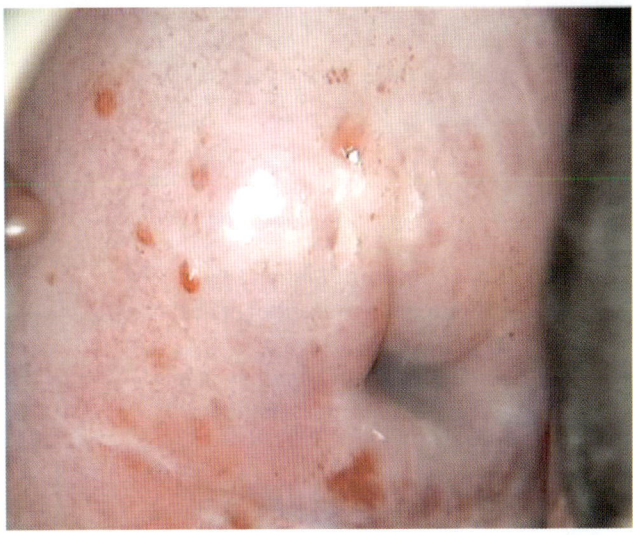

Figure 13-42: Unsatisfactory colposcopy—SCJ not visible

66 A Practical Approach to Cervical Cancer Screening Techniques

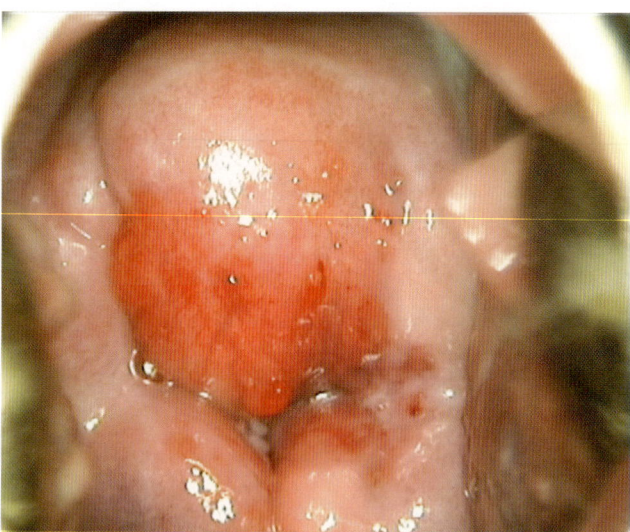

Figure 13-43: Unsatisfactory colposcopy—SCJ not visible in the posterior lip and lateral aspects

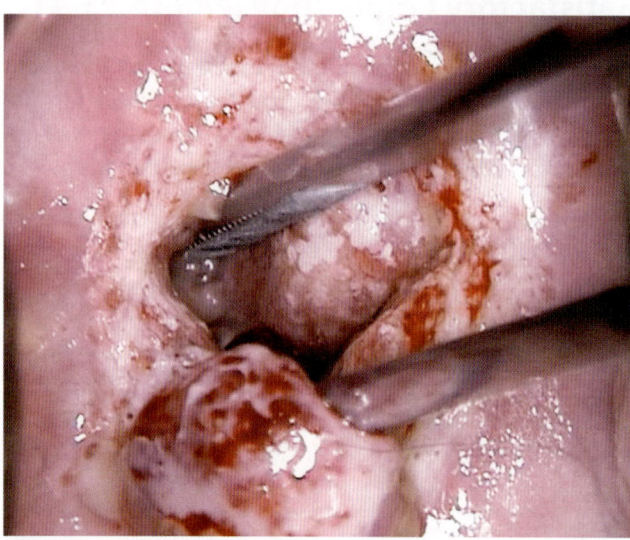

Figure 13-44: Kogan's endocervical speculum

Unsatisfactory colposcopy is seen in:
1. Lesions extending into the endocervical canal
2. In postmenopausal women.
   - Pretreatment with estrogen may help
   - An endocervical curette is mandatory
3. Following conization:
   - SCJ is distorted due to scarring
   - Endocervical curetting is important
4. Following cryo:
   - SCJ will not be visible in 15–20% of the cases

Measures to Overcome Unsatisfactory Colposcopy

- Give pressure on the posterior lip of cervix with a small cotton tip bud to expose the endocervical canal
- Use Kogan's endocervical speculum to open the endocervical canal (Figure 13-44).

> If the entire squamocolumnar junction or the limits of all lesions cannot be completely visualized, a diagnostic cone is necessary

Documentation of Colposcopic Findings

1. Name
2. Age
3. Date of examination
4. Indication for referral
5. Symptoms
6. Clinical finding
7. Colposcopic findings:
   - Colposcopy satisfactory—yes/no
   - SCJ visualized—yes/no
   - Acetowhite epithelium—absent/faint/dense
   - Punctation—absent/fine/coarse
   - Mosaic—absent/fine/coarse
   - Surface—smooth/uneven/nodular
   - Leukoplakia—absent/present
   - Atypical vessels—absent/present
   - Iodine staining—positive/negative
   - Others—inflammation/atrophy/condyloma/papilloma/others.
8. Colposcopic diagnosis:
   - Normal
   - Infection
   - Low-grade SIL
   - High-grade SIL
   - Unsatisfactory
   - Invasive lesion
   - Others—specify
   - HPV

Document the finding diagrammatically on the picture of cervix **(Figure 13-45)**.

COLPOSCOPIC GRADING OF LESIONS

There is considerable overlap of abnormal colposcopic findings in benign conditions, precancerous and cancerous lesions of the cervix. Except the atypical vessels, other abnormal colposcopic findings are not characteristic of

Interpretations of Colposcopy Findings 67

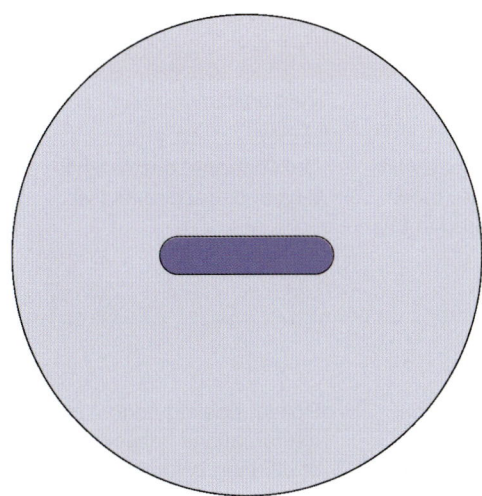

Figure 13-45: External os of cervix

CIN lesions or invasive carcinoma. The primary objective of a colposcopist is to distinguish normal epithelium from abnormal epithelium as well as to differentiate low-grade lesion from a high-grade lesion. It is imperative that at the end of the examination, one arrives at a colposcopic impression of the condition, which will help in the management plan.

One of the important limitations encountered in colposcopic examination is the failure to follow standard diagnostic protocols. Manier times, colposcopic impression of the condition is derived by simple guess or by using a single colposcopic sign. This will jeopardize an accurate correlation with cytologic and histologic results, which may adversely affect management plans.

Therefore, in order to make the colposcopic assessment more objective, reproducible and which will be a meaningful guide to the histological severity of a lesion, several assessment and grading systems are used. These are:
- Coppleson's grading of colposcopic findings
- Reid's colposcopic assessment system (RCI).

Coppleson's Grading of Colposcopic Findings[57]

Grade I: Insignificant—not suspicious
    Minimal neoplastic potential
    Acetowhite epithelium, usually shiny
    Borders are not necessarily sharp
    With or without fine caliber vessels
    Absence of atypical vessels
- The above findings may suggest normal to CIN lesions
- They may be mature or immature metaplastic epithelium, subclinical papilloma virus infection (SPI), CIN I lesions

Grade II: Suspicious lesions
    Lesions have neoplastic potential
    Stromal invasion is not imminent
    Acetowhite epithelium of greater opacity
    Sharp borders
    Dilated regularly shaped vessels with defined pattern
    Absence of atypical vessels
    Increased intercapillary distance
- Lesions correspond from CIN II to CIN III lesions.

Grade III: Highly significant and highly suspicious
    Lesions of high neoplastic potential
    Invasion is imminent
    Very white or gray white epithelium
    Sharp borders
    Dilated irregularly shaped vessels
    Occasional atypical vessels
    Increased intercapillary distance
    Irregular surface contour
- Lesions correspond to CIN III and early invasion can be anticipated.

Reid's Colposcopic Assessment System (RCI)[58,59]

RCI is a systematic, objective method of colposcopically grading the severity of premalignant cervical disease. It provides a means of standardizing the evaluation of cervical disease.

RCI was developed by Reid et al. in 1984. The original RCI used five objective colposcopic signs, namely:
- Lesion margin
- Thickness of tissue
- Color of acetowhitening
- Nature of blood vessels
- Iodine staining

The modified RCI includes only four colposcopic signs and thickness is not included in the assessment **(Table 13-1)**.

In Reid's colposcopic assessment system, four unique colposcopy signs are used:
1. Lesion margin
2. Acetowhite reaction
3. Vascular pattern, and
4. Iodine staining.

The first three signs are evaluated following application of 5% acetic acid. The fourth sign, iodine reaction is evaluated after application of one quarter Lugol's iodine.

Each of the above colposcopic signs is divided into three objective categories. Depending upon the severity of the lesion, each category is assigned a score of 0, 1 or 2.

A Practical Approach to Cervical Cancer Screening Techniques

Table 13-1: The Modified Reid Colposcopic Index Colposcopic grading performed with 5% aqueous acetic acid and Lugol's iodine solution

Colposcopic signs	Zero point	One point	Two points
Color	Less intense acetowhitening (not completely opaque); indistinct acetowhitening; semi-translucent acetowhitening; acetowhitening beyond the margin of the transformation zone. Pure snow-white color with prominent surface seen.	Intermediate shade—grey/white color and shiny surface (most lesions should be scored in this category)	Dull, opaque, oyster white, grey, loss of surface reflectivity
Lesion margin and surface configuration	Flat lesions with indistinct margins. Feathered or finely scalloped margins. Angular, jagged lesions. Satellite lesions beyond the margin of the transformation zone.	Regular-shaped, symmetrical lesions with smooth, sharp, straight outlines	Rolled, peeling edges, internal demarcations between areas of differing colposcopic appearance—a central area of high-grade change and peripheral area of low-grade change.
Vessels	Fine/Uniform-caliber vessels—closely placed. Ill-defined areas of fine punctuation and/or mosaic pattern vessels beyond the margin of the transformation zone.	Absence of surface vessels following acetic acid application	Coarse punctation or mosaic, individual vessel dilated, arranged in sharply demarcated well-defined pattern.
Iodine staining	Positive iodine uptake giving mahogany-brown color. Negative uptake of insignificant lesion, i.e. yellow staining by a lesion scoring three points or less on the first three criteria • Areas beyond the margin of the transformation zone.	Partial iodine uptake-variegated, speckled appearance or 'tortoise shell appearance'	Negative iodine uptake of significant lesion, i.e. yellow staining by a lesion already scoring four points or more on the first three criteria'

- 0 point represents benign changes of HPV infection or mild dysplasia (low-grade lesion)
- 1 point is indicative of CIN I or CIN II (intermediate-grade lesion)
- 2 points is indicative of CIN II or CIN III (high-grade lesion).

I. Lesion Margin

Defines the character of the margin of a lesion
0 points (Low grade lesion)
'0' points are given to lesions whose margins are irregular, flocculated and feathered like. Some lesions are angular, map like lesions also called geographic lesions. Satellite lesions are seen outside the TZ, are given 0 points. Condyloma like lesions (micropapilliferous) are also low grade lesions.

The following lesions are given a score of '0' **(Figures 13-46A to D).**

'1' Point (Intermediate Lesions) (Figure 13-47)

A score of 1 is given to a lesion whose margins are smooth and have straight border.

'2' Points (High-grade Lesions) (Figure 13-48)

Lesions which are raised with peeling edges are given a score of 2.

In high-grade lesions, the cell-to-cell cohesiveness is so fragile that the epithelial edges tend to detach and peel off from the underlying stroma, presenting as rolled edges. This can be demonstrated by gently pushing away the tissue with a cotton swab. Theses are seen exclusively at the new SCJ.

High-grade lesion may also show internal demarcation (internal margin) between two different grades of lesions with a minor lesion in the periphery with central area showing high-grade lesion **(Figure 13-49)**.

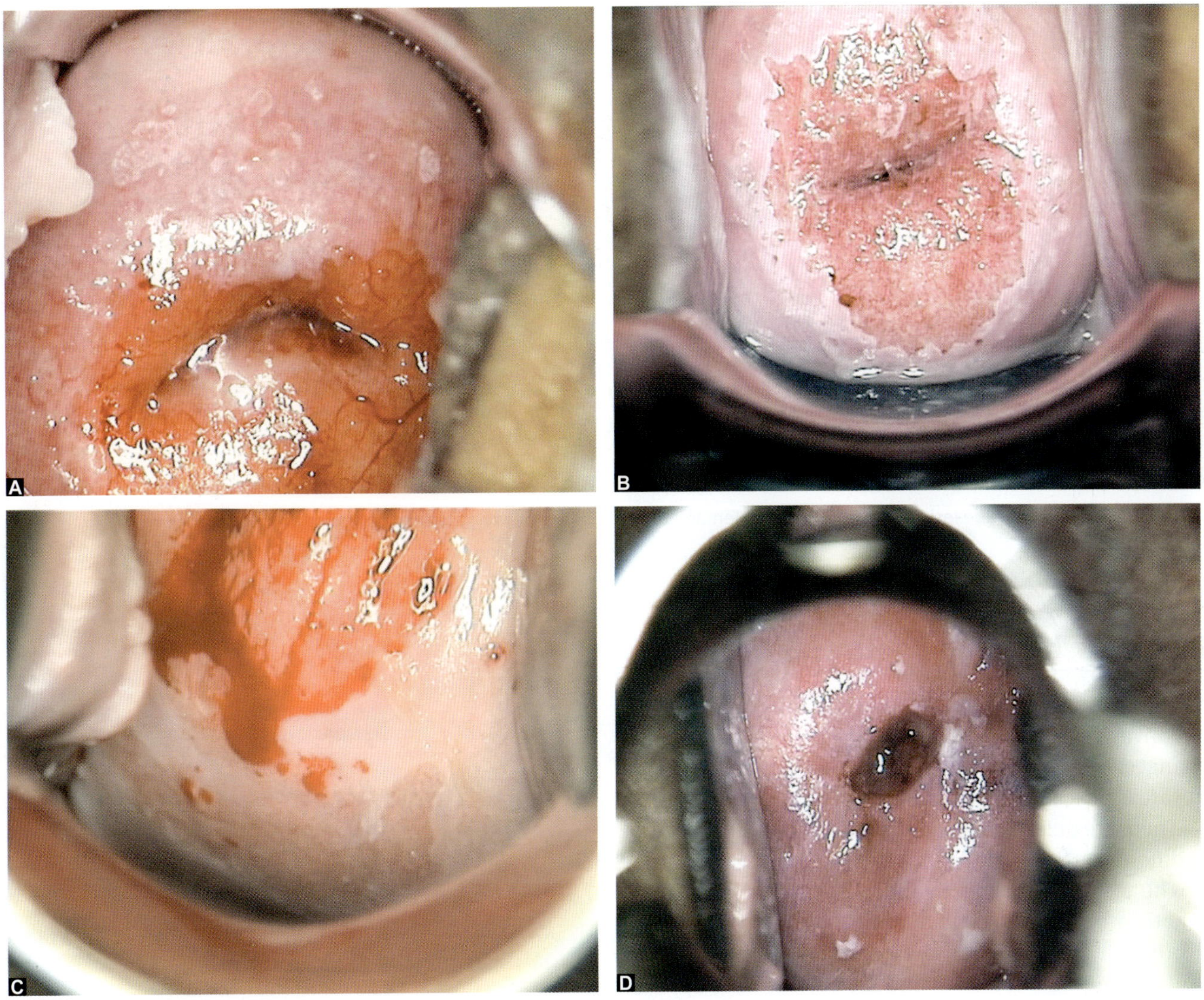

Interpretations of Colposcopy Findings

Figures 13-46A to D: Scoring of lesion margin. Score '0'. A. Satellite lesions; B. Lesion with scalloped margin; C. Geographic map-like lesion; D. Lesions suggesting condylomas

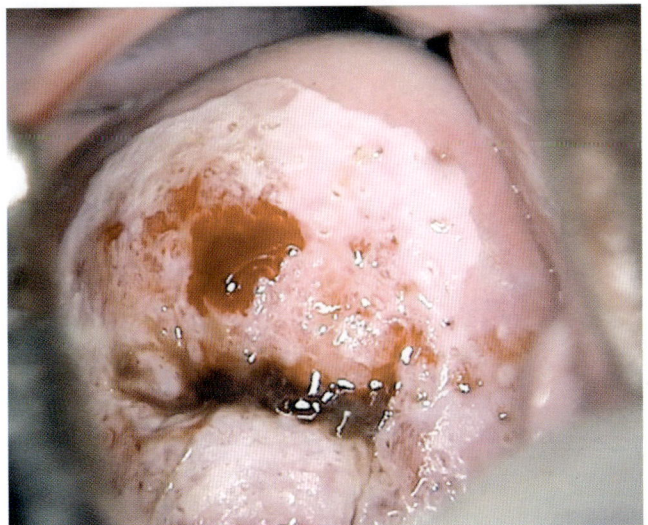

Figure 13-47: Lesion with straight border

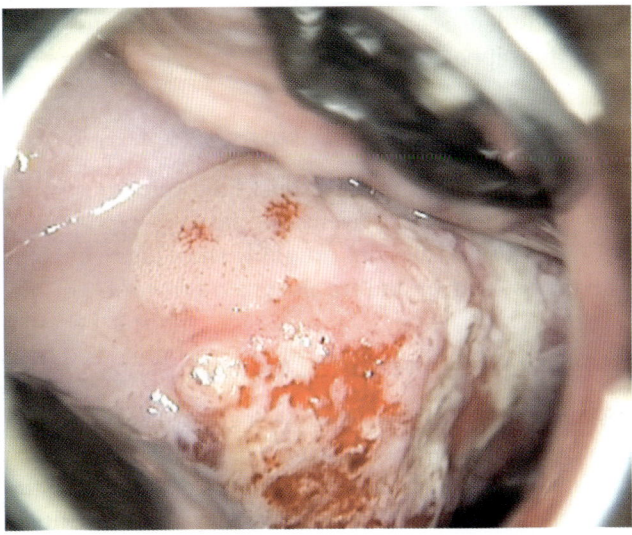

Figure 13-48: High-grade lesion with peeling edges

70 A Practical Approach to Cervical Cancer Screening Techniques

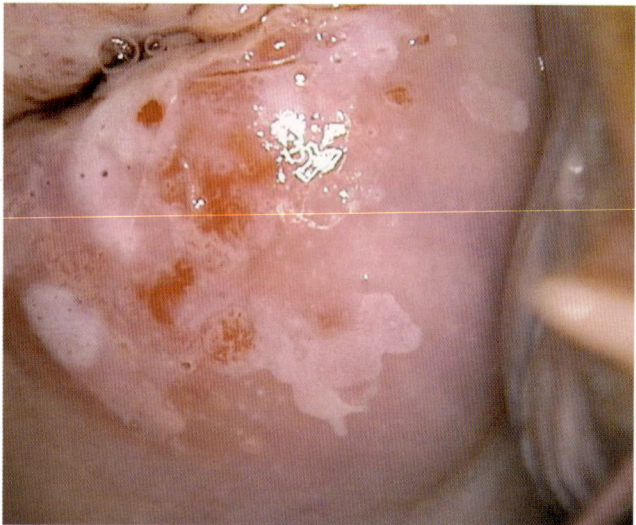

Figure 13-49: High-grade lesion showing internal demarcation

II. Acetowhitening (Figure 13-50)

Normal squamous metaplasia, different grades of CIN and invasive cancers exhibit varying grades of acetowhite changes. Less experienced colposlopist may recognize all the areas of acetowhite changes as abnormal.

There are different mechanisms for acetowhite reaction in different grades of lesions.

The acetowhite change in minor lesion is due to transient reaction between acetic acid and abnormal envelop protein in HPV-infected keratinocytes. Therefore, the acetowhitening is transient and the color change appears and disappears quickly.

The acetowhite change seen in high-grade lesion is due to osmotic dehydration, which accentuates the high content of optically dense chronatin in CIN 3. It takes time to get the acetowhite appearance, but remains longer.

'0' Point (Low-Grade Lesions)

Low-grade lesions exhibit indistinct, faint, semitransparent acetowhitening and are given '0' point.

Condylamatous lesions are shiny snow-white in color with intense surface and are also given a score of '0'.

'1' Point (Intermediate Lesions)

Lesions which are shiny, off white or gray white in color are given a score of 1.

Here, in deeper layers, there is light absorption by the atypical nuclei, whereas the upper layers with cellular maturation reflect the light from the surface.

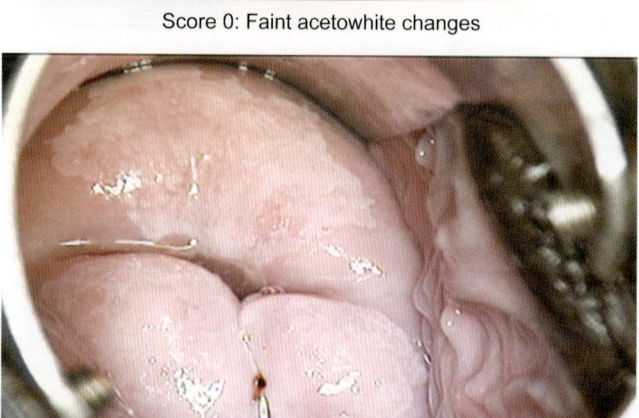

Score 0: Faint acetowhite changes

Score 1: Shiny gray white

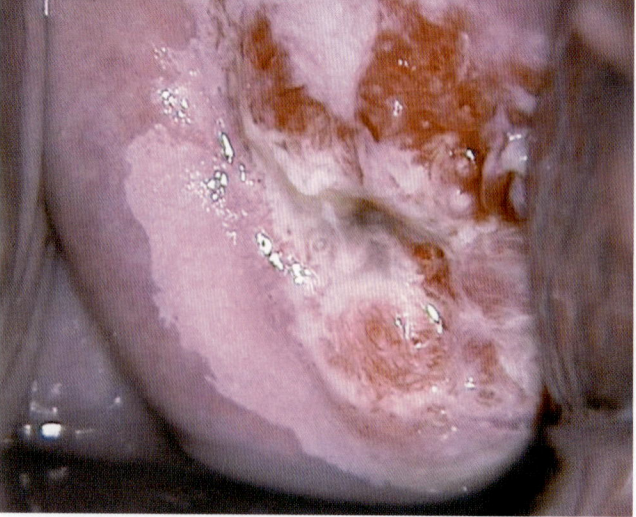

Score 2: Dense acetowhite changes

Figure 13-50: Comparative pictures showing acetowhite changes in different grades of lesions

'2' Points (High-grade Lesions)

Lesions which are dirty oyster gray in color and dense acetowhite in appearance are given a score of 2. In these lesions, there is intense light absorption by the chromatin dense nuclei and there is no light reflection from the surface due to paucity of cytoplasm in the superficial epithelial cells.

III. Vascular Pattern

Vascular pattern describes fine/coarse punctation, mosaics and atypical vessels.

Prominent vascular changes are often seen in nonspecific and HPV infection due to proliferative changes. Mosaics and punctation within the TZ are more likely to represent CIN and outside TZ are less likely to represent CIN.

'0' Point (Low-grade Lesions) (Figures 13-51A and B)

A score of '0' is given to a lesion where fine caliber vessels and nondilated capillary loops are seen. There may also be ill-defined areas of fine punctation and mosaics. The vessels arborize like branches of a tree and they become thin as they branch at distally.

'1' Point (Intermediate Lesions) (Figure 13-52)

A score of 1 given to a lesion which is devoid of superficial vessels. This is due to gradual compression and depression of the normal capillary looped vessels within the nuclear dense tissue, preventing tem from being visualized.

'2' Point (High-grade Lesions) (Figures 13-53 to 13-55)

A score of 2 is given to a lesion with coarsely dilated vessels, arranged in well-defined sharply demarcated pattern, coarse punctation, mosaics and atypical vessels.

The vascular changes are due to angiogenesis, new vessels feeding a neoplasm.

Following application of acetic acid, the scores of the first three colposcopic signs are added up to get a preliminary score.

When iodine is applied to the cervix, not only CIN lesions, but also normal tissues biopsy sites, vaginitis, cervicitis and atropic tissue will also reject iodine staining; therefore, it appears mustard yellow.

Therefore, the score of the first three colposcopy signs will influence the score of the last colposcopy sign, namely iodine staining.

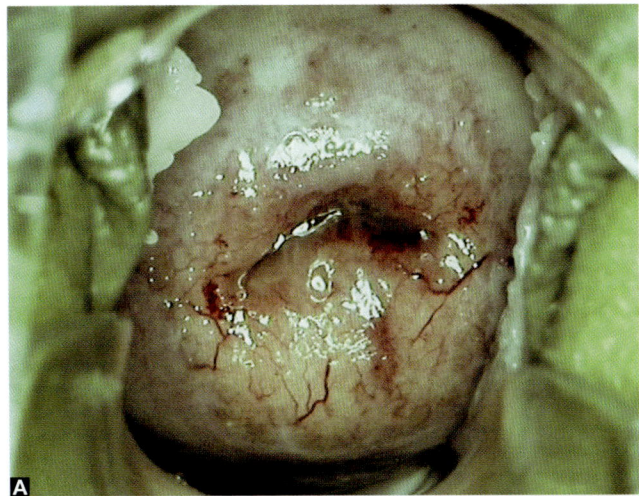
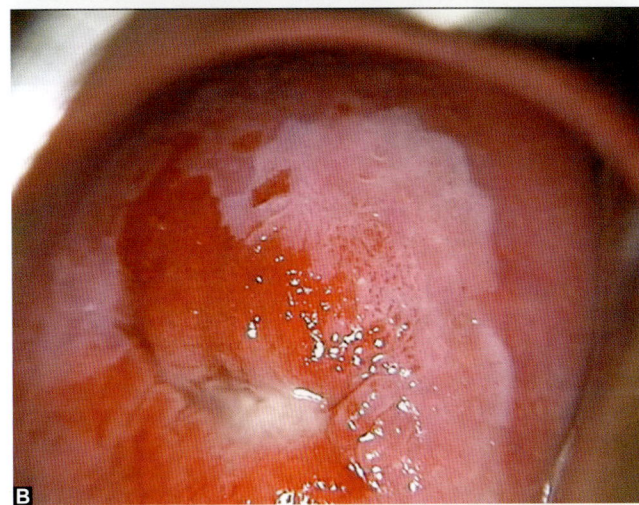

Figures 13-51A and B: A. Lesion showing arborizing; B. Lesion showing fine punctation, fine caliber vessels

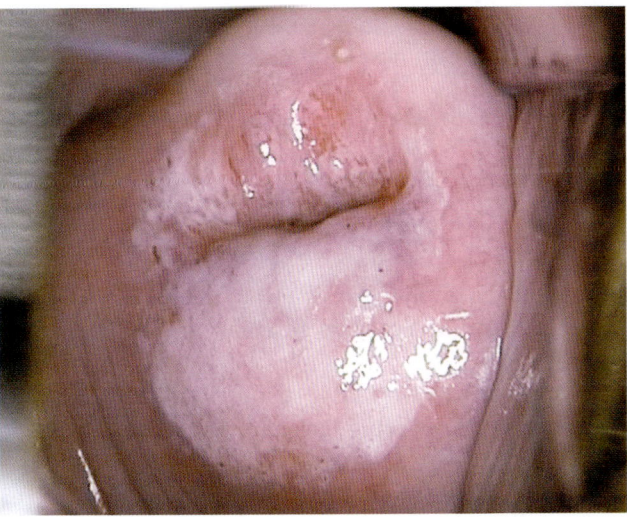

Figure 13-52: Lesion which is devoid of vessels

72 A Practical Approach to Cervical Cancer Screening Techniques

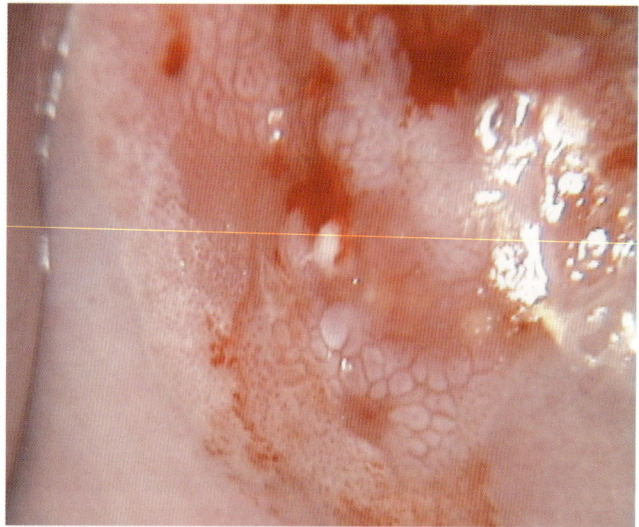

Figure 13-53: Lesion showing coarse mosaics and punctation

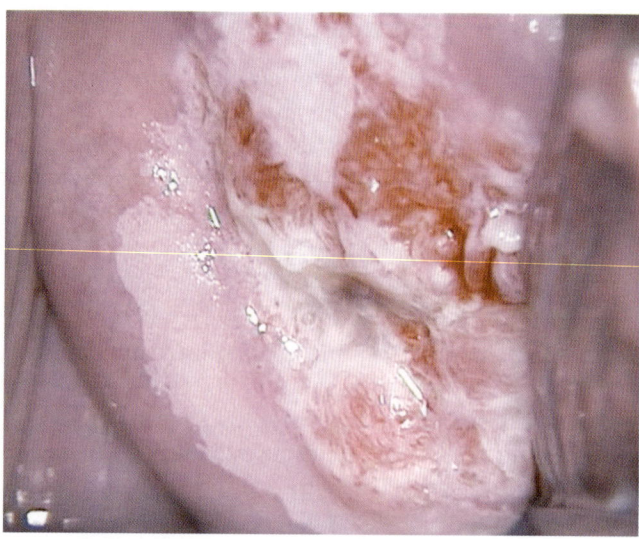

Figure 13-55: Atypical vessels

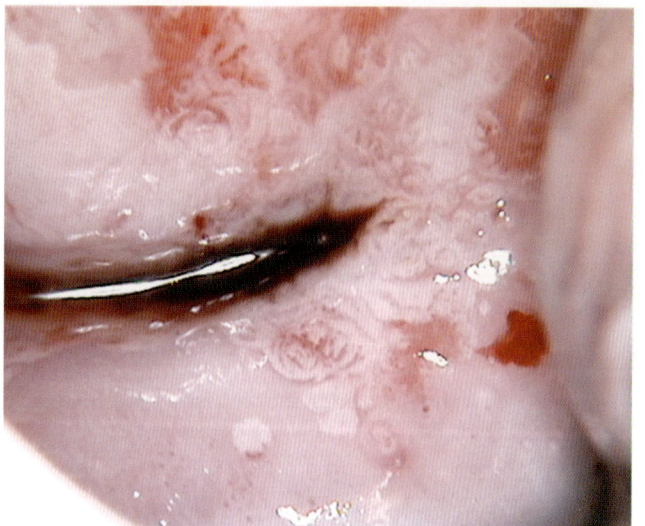

Figure 13-54: Lesion showing coarsely dilated vessels with mosaics

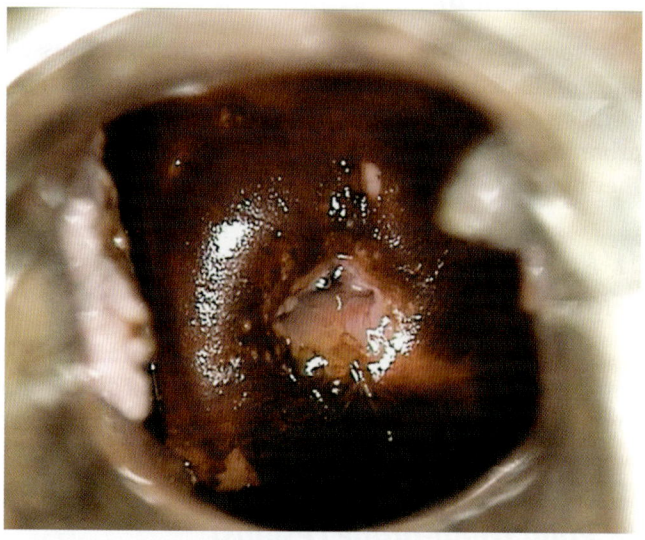

Figure 13-56: Normal squamous epithelium with mahogany brown coloration—Score '0'

IV. Iodine Staining

'0' point

A score of '0' is given to a lesion which shows:
- Positive iodine reaction showing mahogany brown coloration.
- Lesion which rejects iodine staining, but the preliminary score was 2 or less (may be columnar cells, metaplastic cells, etc).

A score of '0' is given to the following lesions **(Figures 13-56 and 13-57)**.

'1' Point (Figure 13-58)

A score of 1 is given to a lesion which shows partial iodine uptake with stained and unstained areas—tortoise shell appearance.

'2' Points

A score of 2 is given to a lesion which rejects iodine and the preliminary score has 3 or more **(Figure 13-59)**.

The total RCI score is determined by adding the four individual colposcopy signs **(Figure 13-60)**.

Interpretations of Colposcopy Findings 73

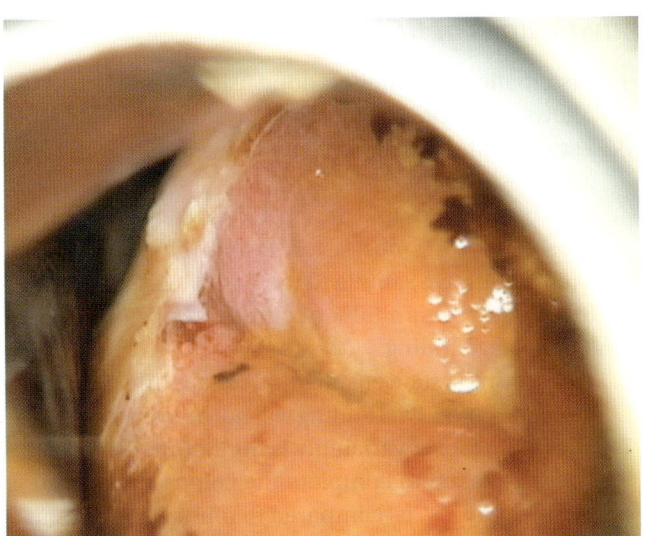

Figure 13-57: The lesion rejects iodine and stains yellow, but the preliminary score was less than 2—Score '0'

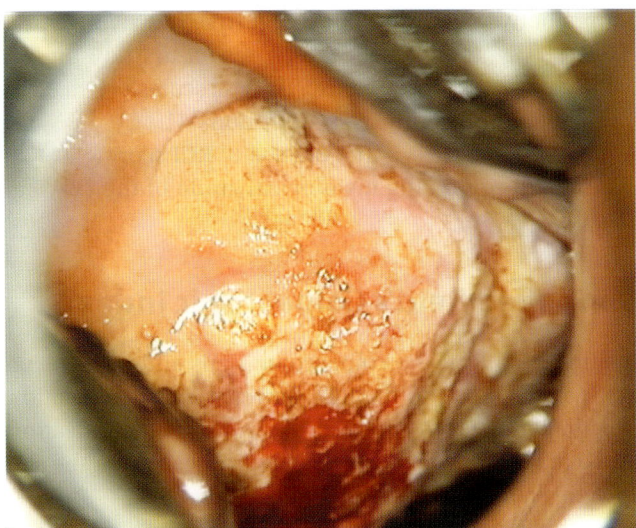

Figure 13-59: Lesion with a preliminary score of 6 with iodine negative areas—Score '2'

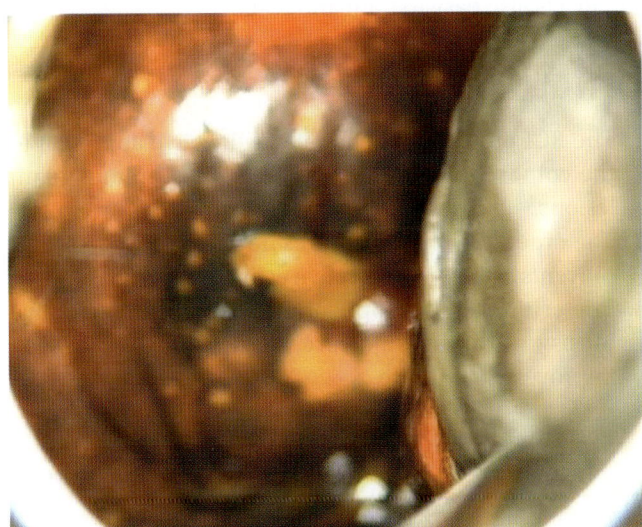

Figure 13-58: Iodine uptake and iodine negative areas—Score '1'

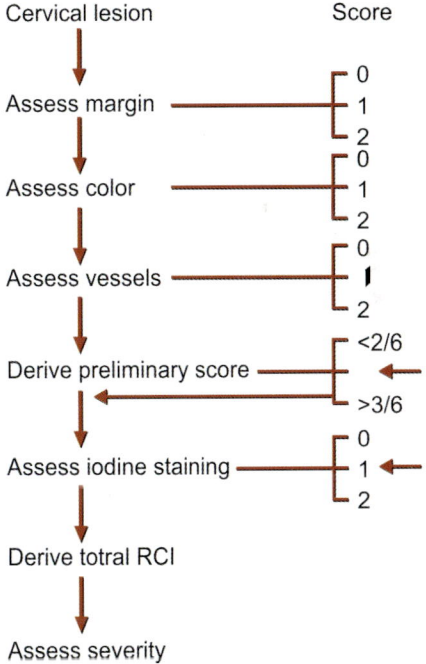

Figure 13-60: Flow chart to determine RCI score

The RCI is always represented as a ratio
The denominator is always 8
The numerator is the sum of the four colposcopy signs score
They are reported as 2/8, 6/8, etc.
The RCI score is then correlated with the clinical diagnosis.

The RCI Clinical Correlation (Table 13-2)

The total RCI score represents a weighted scoring system predictive of the severity of premalignant cervical lesions.

Table 13-2: The RCI clinical correlation	
Numerator	Indicative of Score
0–2	HPV or CIN I (Low grade)
3–5	CIN I or CIN II (Intermediate grade)
6–8	CIN II or CIN III (High grade)

In general, the lower the RCI score, the less serious is the degree of disease. Numerator scores between zero and two are predictive of CIN I or human papilloma virus infection.

74 A Practical Approach to Cervical Cancer Screening Techniques

Scores between 3 and 5 are suggestive of CIN I or CIN II. Generally, total scores of 3 represent mild dysplasia, while scores of 5 represent CIN II. Total scores of 6 to 8 are predictive of moderate-to-severe lesion.

Studies have shown that the use of RCI scoring is 97% accurate in predicting histological grade of the cervical disease.

Simplified Reid's Colposcopic Index

In simplified RCI; the colposcopic signs and the scoring system are similar to the RCI; however, site specification is an integral part in reporting of results. Site specification is useful for the follow-up of patients as well as for the site specific management of low-grade lesions.

In this assessment system, the cervix is divided into 4 quadrants by an imaginary line passing through the cervix from 9 o'clock to 3 o'clock and from 12 o'clock to 6 o'clock position. Examination of each quadrant is done in a clockwise direction starting from the right upper (RU) quadrant **(Figure 13-61)**.

Colposcopy signs and scoring system are similar to the RCI.[59,60]

Reporting of Simplified RCI (Figure 13-62)

Reporting is done as shown in the figure, which shows a lesion with a score of 1, involving right upper quadrant (RU) and left upper quadrant (LU); therefore, it is reported as RU LURCI 1.

Advantages of RCI

1. Systematic assessment is done using specific criteria.
2. Allows differentiation of normal from abnormal tissue.
3. Permits differentiation of low-grade lesion from high-grade lesion.
4. Even in a large complex lesion, biopsy can be taken from the site, showing most severe lesion, thereby providing a representative sample to the pathologist.
5. RCI is more than 90% accurate in predicting the histological finding.
6. This scoring system ensures that serious disease will not be missed and trivial finding will not be overinterpreted.
7. The interobsever variability is minimum.
8. The time taken to complete the colposcopy record is significantly less as compared to routine conventional colposcopy, where the results are recorded as hand drawings.
9. As the colposcopy is given as a score, it is easy to compare with previous findings during follow-up visits.
10. RCI is also easy to train and teach.

CONCLUSION

1. The RCI provides a systematic, subjective approach to the colposcopic assessment of cervical premalignant lesions.
2. The orderly method reassures novice colposcopist and prevents arbitrary, subjective estimates.
3. The critical colposcopic appraisal helps in selective biopsy of the most severe cervical disease, which improves patient care.

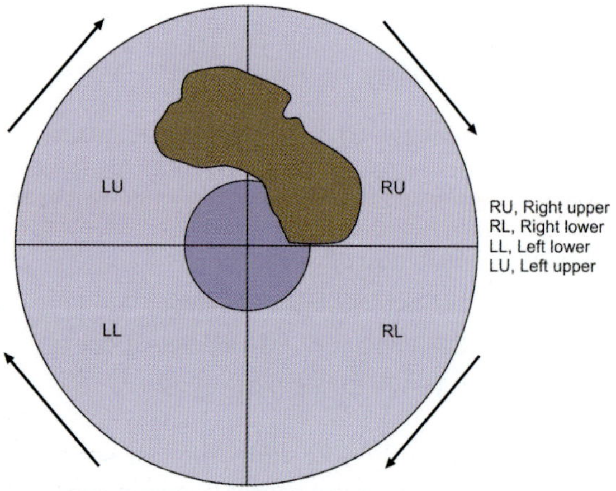

Figure 13-61: Simplified Reid's colposcopic index

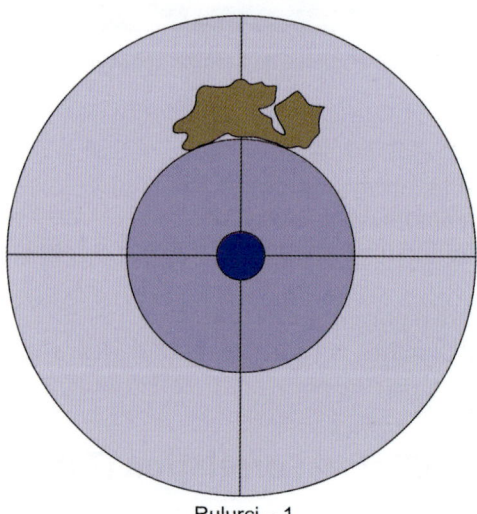

Figure 13-62: Reporting of simplified RCI

> Any abnormal area must be biopsied and confirmed by biopsy
> Any temptation to make a histological diagnosis based on colposcopic findings should be resisted

COLPOSCOPY APPEARANCE OF BENIGN, CIN AND MALIGNANT LESIONS OF THE CERVIX

Ectropion of the Cervix (Figures 13-63A to C)

Ectropion results from eversion of the endocervical epithelium and SCJ onto the portio cervix. When seen with naked eye, ectropion is velvety red in appearance due to the reflection from the underlying stromal vessels. Because of the mucus content, there is transient faint acetowhite change when acetic acid is applied. This change reverts to normal quickly. Columar epithelium does not stain with iodine due to lack of glycogen. There may be varying degrees of metaplasia as well. The ectropion is markedly seen in the adolescence, first pregnancy and with oral contraceptive use.

Colposcopic Appearance of Metaplasia (Figures 13-64 to 13-67)

- Acetowhite changes are faint and transient
- Acetowhite satellite lesions may be seen away from the SCJ
- The gland openings may be surrounded by metaplastic epithelium
- The margins are irregular and indistinct from the normal epithelium
- Prominent normal arborizing vessels may be seen
- The metaplastic epithelium is iodine negative.

Nabothian Cyst (Figures 13-68 to 13-70)

The nabothian cysts appear yellow and translucent. There can be multiple nabothian cysts.

The endocervical gland crypts get occluded due to squamous metaplasia, resulting in distension and cyst formation. The nabothian cyst appears translucent with increased vascularity over the surface which are normal branching vessels. The nabothian cysts are seen in the area of TZ.

Endocervical Polyps (Figures 13-71A and B)

Focal hyperplasia of the endocervical epithelium and the stroma result in polyp formation and they protrude through

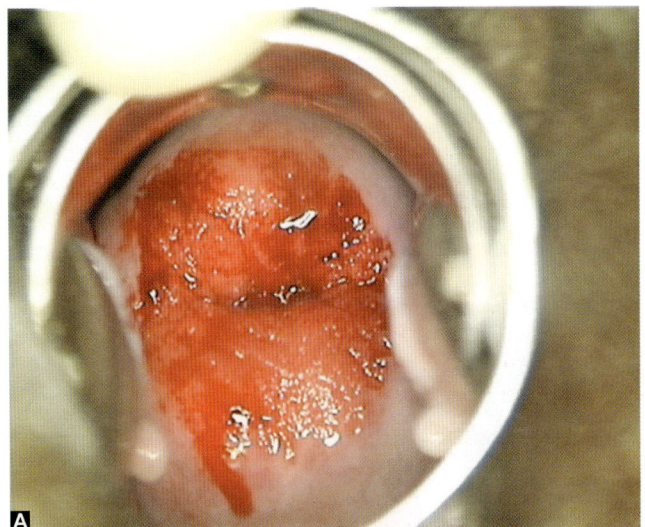
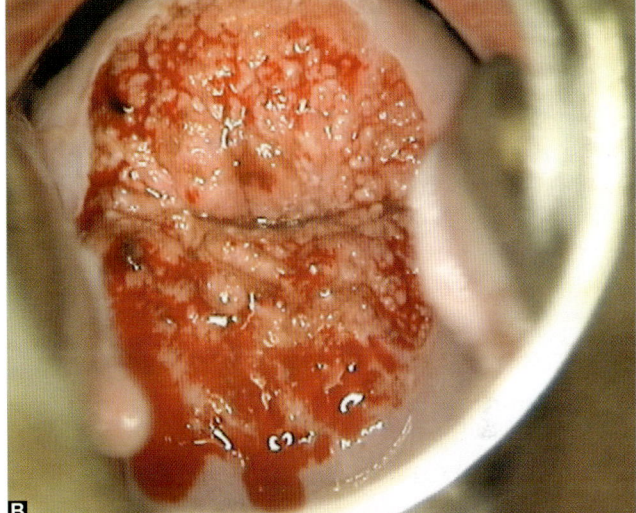
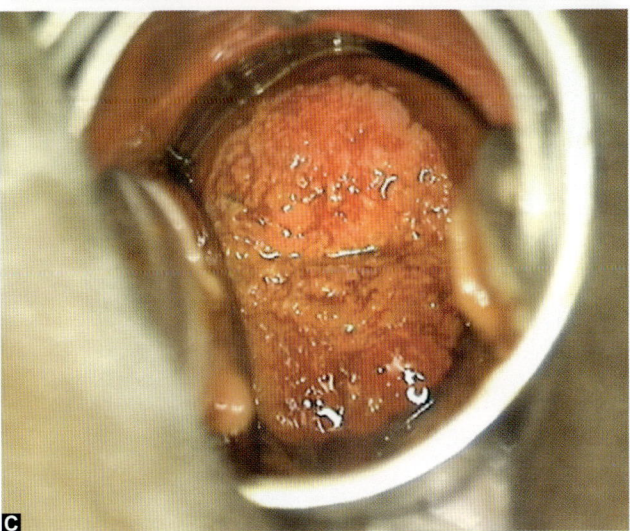

Figures 13-63A to C: Ectropion of the cervix. A. Large ectropion of the cervix; B. The columnar epithelium is more prominent after acetic acid application; C. The columnar epithelium does not take up iodine

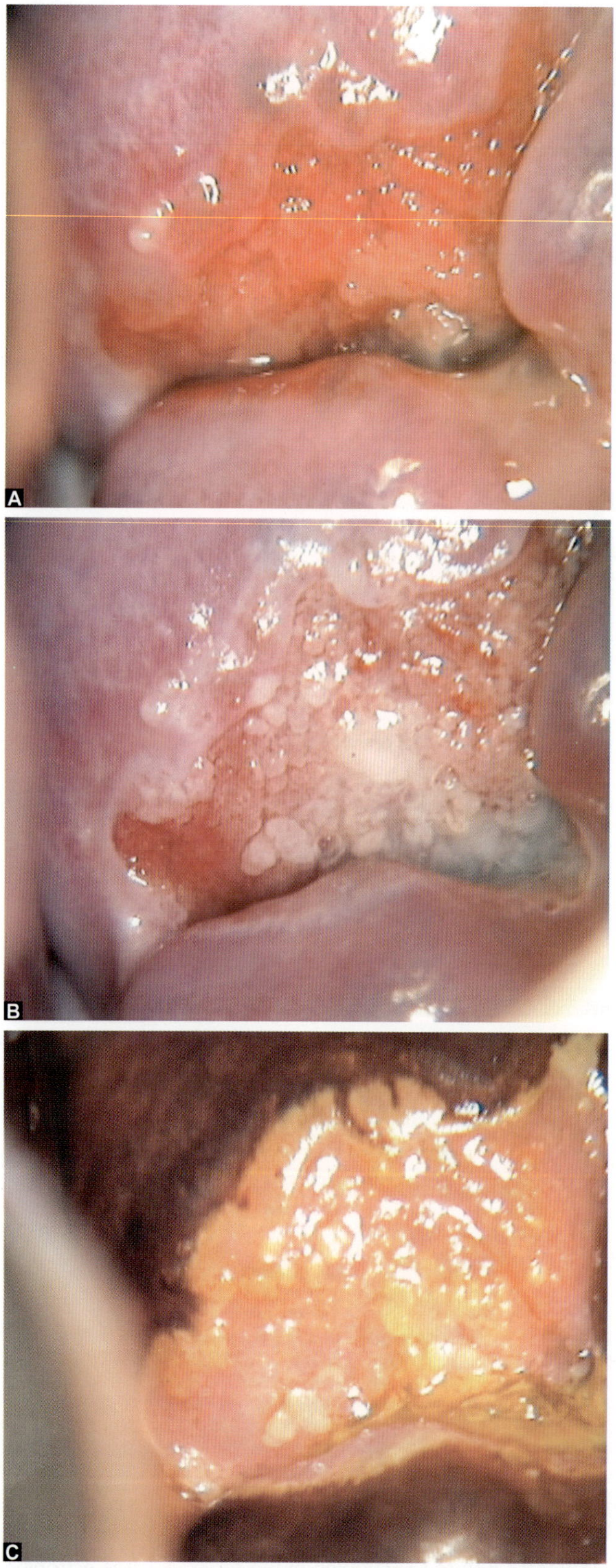

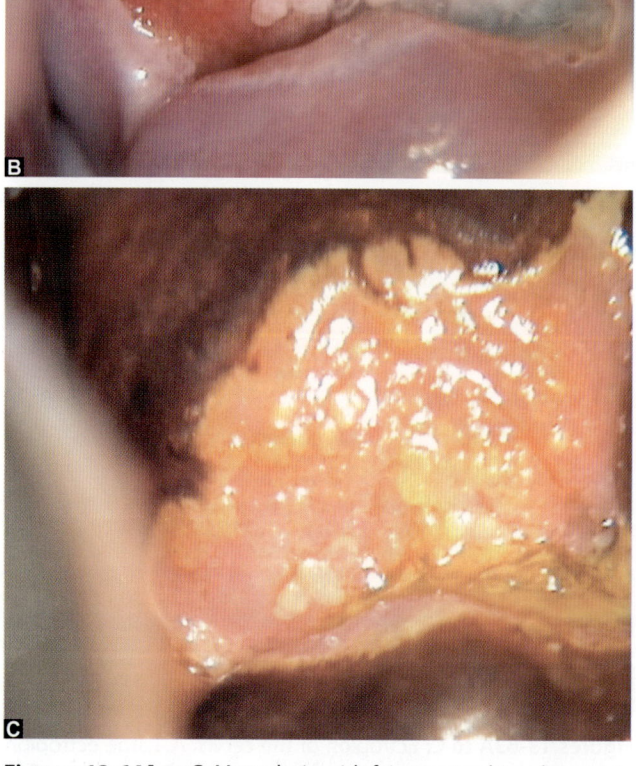

Figures 13-64A to C: Metaplasia with faint acetowhite changes in the anterior lip. The SCJ is not fully visualized. The metaplstic area is iodine negative

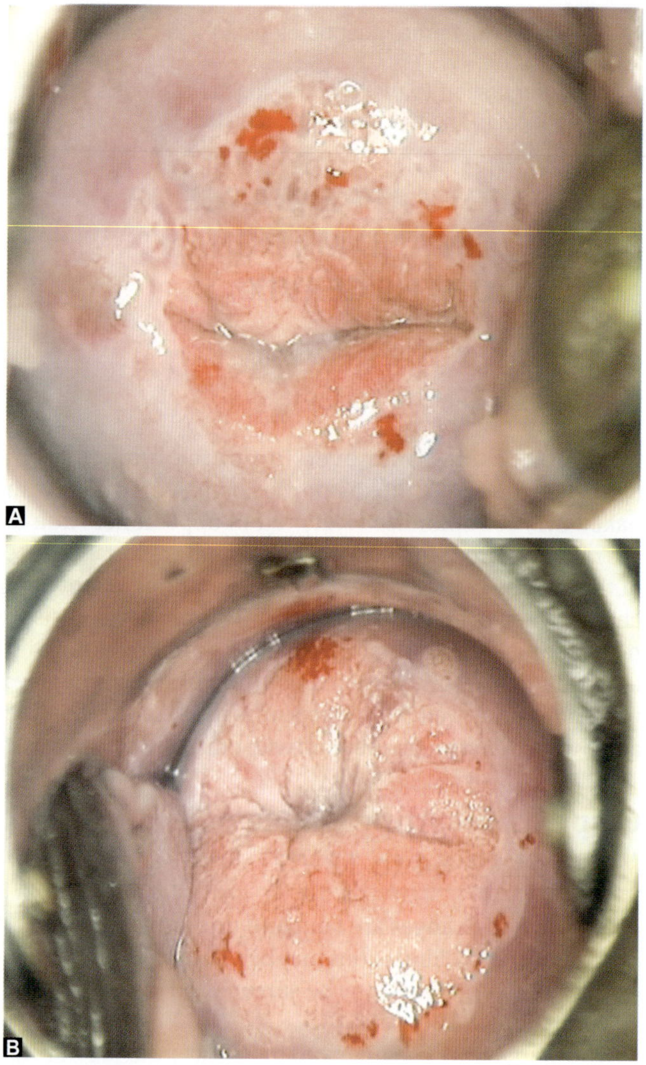

Figures 13-65A and B: A small ectropion with a rim of metaplasia at the periphery. The gland openings are surrounded by metaplastic squamous epithelium. The SCJ is well visulized

the cervical os. There may be increased vascularity and inflammatory changes. Squamous metaplasia may also occur on the surface of the polyp.

Because of the ulceration, patients can present with postcoital bleeding. These polyps should be removed for histopathological examination.

Colposcopy Appearance in Postmenopausal Women (Figures 13-72A to F)

Atrophic Changes

In postmenopausal women, due to the lack of estrogen, the squamous epithelium becomes very thin and brittle. As a result thin branching vessels from the underlying stroma

Interpretations of Colposcopy Findings

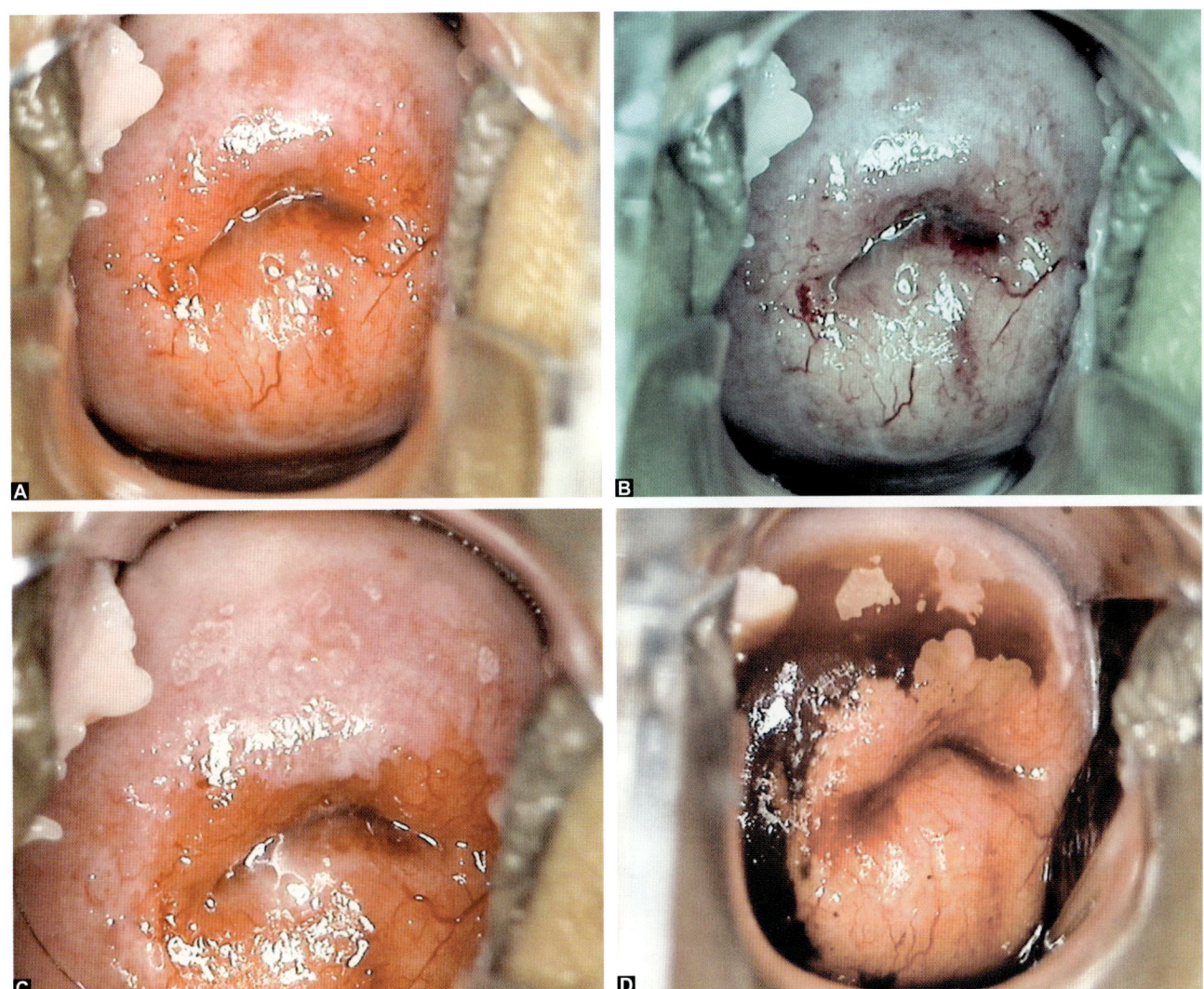

Figures 13-66A to D: A large ectropion with prominent normal arborizing vessels. The vessels are clearly seen through the green filter. There are acetowhite satellite lesions away from the SCJ, which are iodine negative, suggesting HPV infection.

can be easily seen. The tissue also gets easily traumatized and petechial hemorrhages can be seen. The SCJ will be within the endocervical canal and the colposcopy will most often be unsatisfactory. Due to the lack of glycogen, the squamous epithelium does not stain with iodine or partial iodine uptake may be seen.

Infection of the Cervix (Figure 13-73)

Cervicitis may make colposcopy assessment difficult. Due to the dilatation of the underlying stromal vessels, the denuded areas appear red. Infections such as trichomoniasis result in such diffuse erythema of the cervix and vagina and are often called 'strawberry cervix'. In the presence of infection, necessary investigations and treatment should be carried out before the colposcopic assessment.

Colposcopy in Pregnancy (Figures 13-74 and 13-75)

During pregnancy, there are a number of physiological and architectural changes and cytological alterations in the cervix. This makes it difficult in performing colposcopy and interpreting and evaluating the cytology and colposcopy findings. There is significant increase in the cervical volume due to hypertrophy of the fibromuscular tissue, edema and increased vascularity. The increased vascularity induces a bluish hue to the cervix **(Figure 13-74)**. The endocervical canal gets everted exposing the columnar epithelium to the vaginal acidity **(Figure 13-75)**. The eversion of the endocervix is at its maximum by 20 weeks of gestation; therefore, the TZ is fully visualized and the colposcopy is satisfactory in majority of the cases.

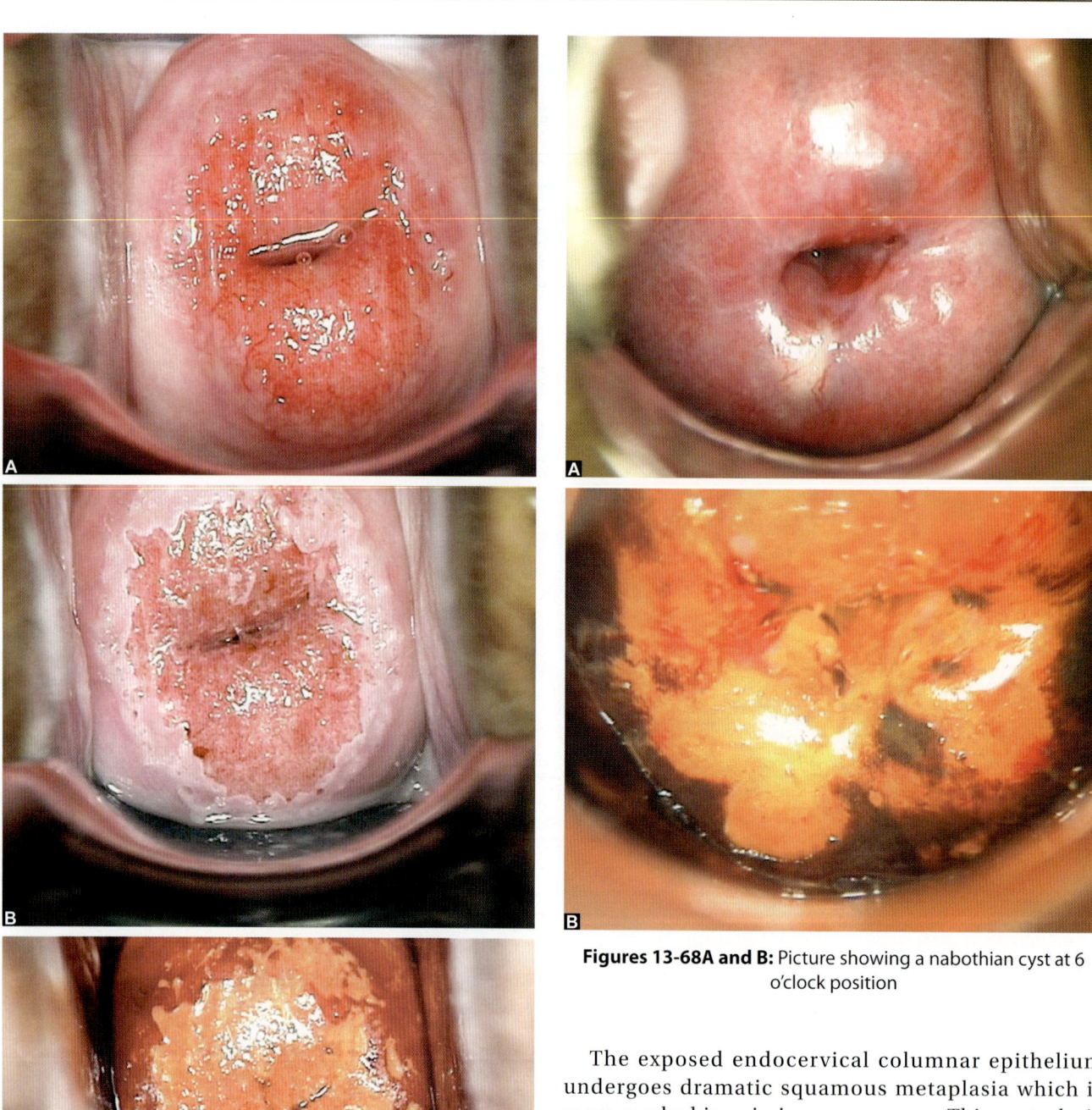

Figures 13-67A to C: A large ectropion with metaplasia at the periphery. The columnar epithelium and the metaplastic areas are iodine negative

Figures 13-68A and B: Picture showing a nabothian cyst at 6 o'clock position

The exposed endocervical columnar epithelium undergoes dramatic squamous metaplasia which is more marked in primiparous women. This metaplasia appears acetowhite after acetic acid application, and this effect is exaggerated by the bluish hue imparted by the increased vascularity of pregnancy. This squamous metaplasia continues until 36 weeks of gestation and the epithelium returns to its endocervical position in the puerperium. Within the metaplastic areas one can also see fine punctuation and mosaic pattern. These changes may result in difficulty in differentiating squamous metaplasia from CIN lesions and may lead to over diagnosis of lesions even by experienced colposcopists. In subsequent pregnancies, there is gaping of the endocervical canal and the squamous metaplasia occurs predominantly later in

Interpretations of Colposcopy Findings

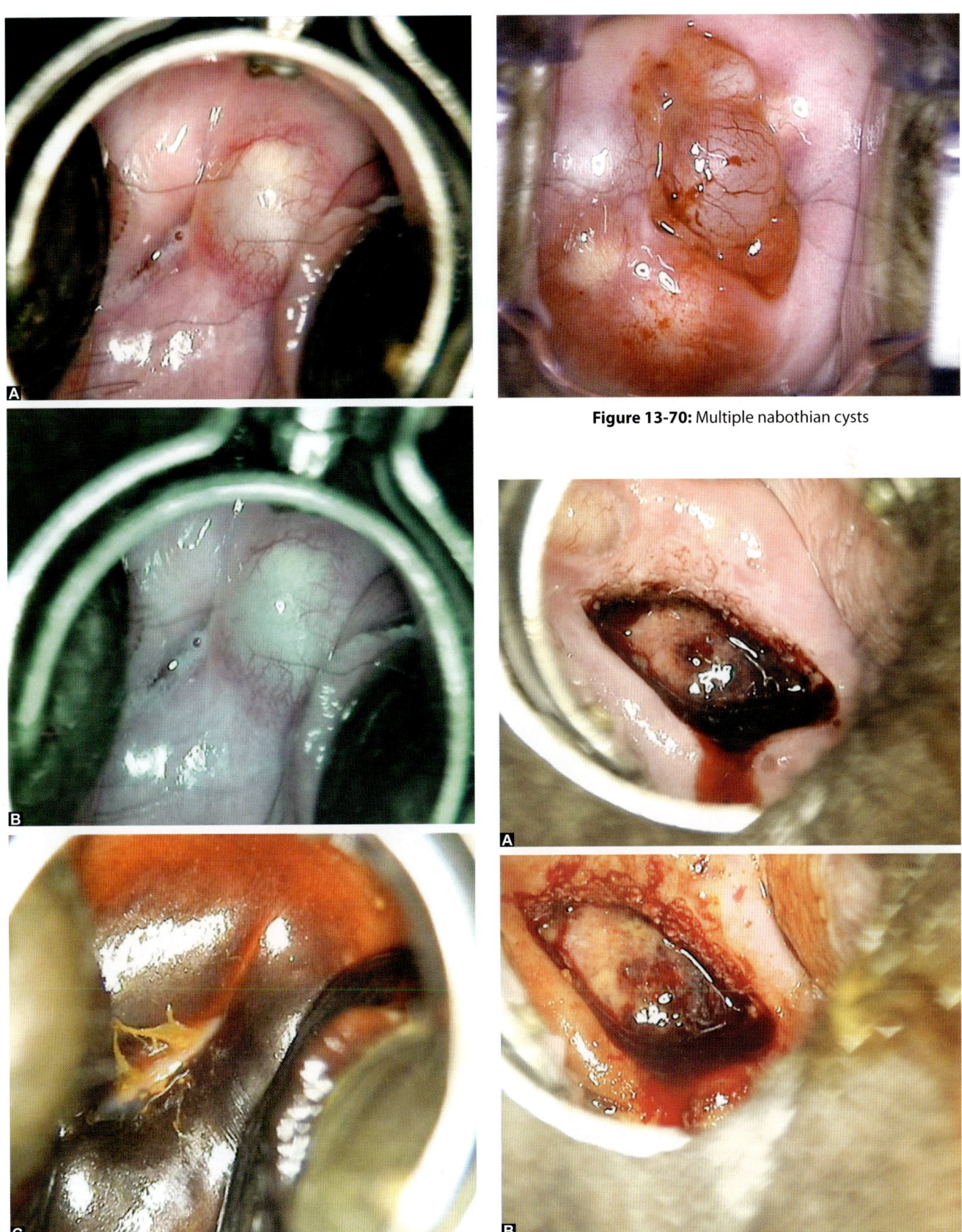

Figures 13-69A to C: Nabothian cyst with increased vascularity on the surface

Figure 13-70: Multiple nabothian cysts

Figures 13-71A and B: Endocervical polyp

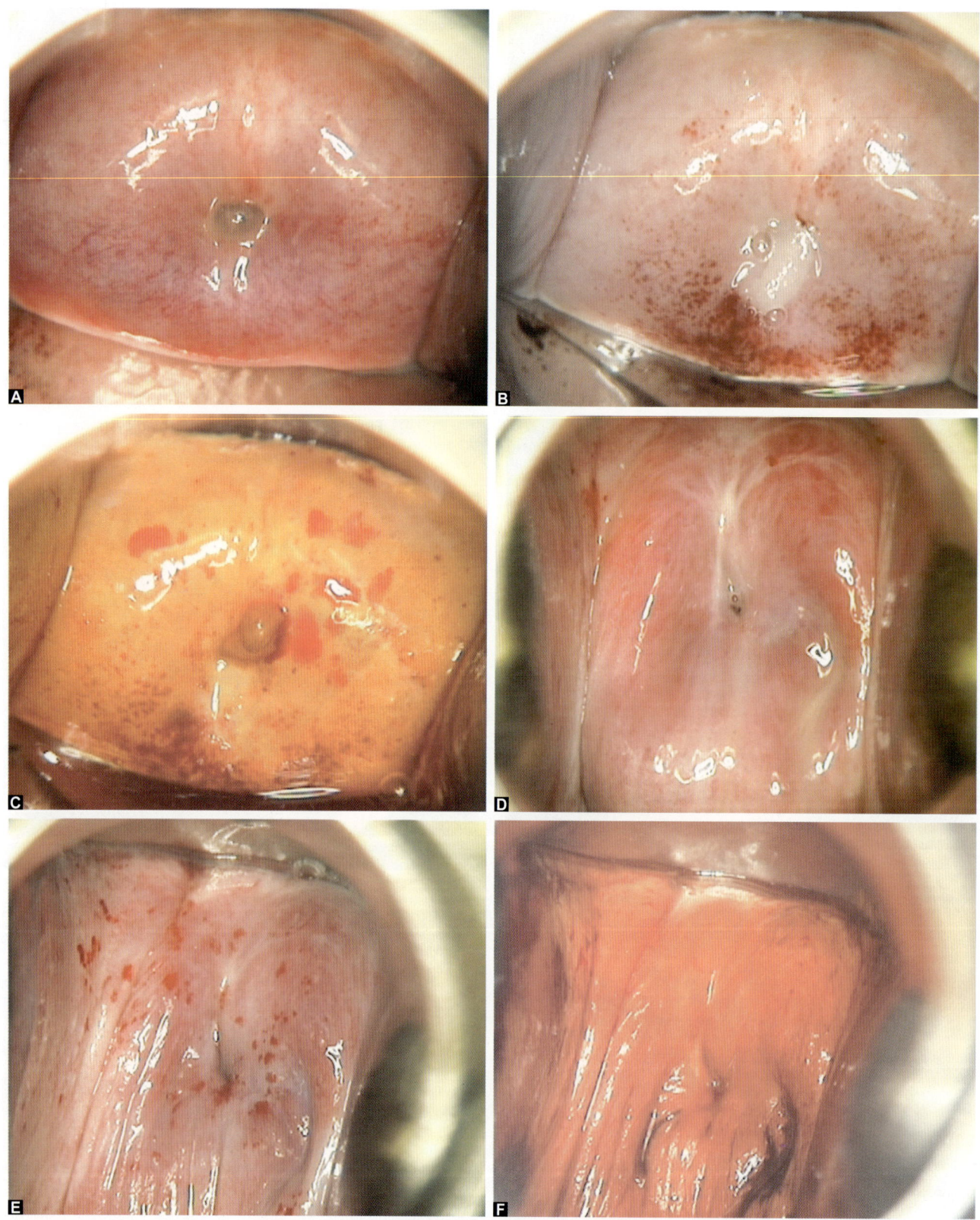

Figures 13-72A to F: Postmenopausal cervix covered by thin atrophic epithelium showing petechial hemorrhages. Due to the loss of glycogen, the atrophic epithelium rejects iodine

Interpretations of Colposcopy Findings 81

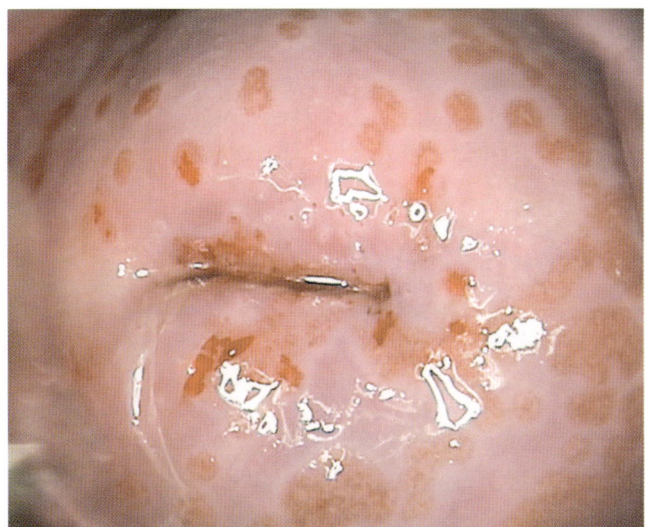

Figure 13-73: Colpitis/cervicitis with patchy areas of denuded squamous epithelium on the portio vaginalis of the cervix

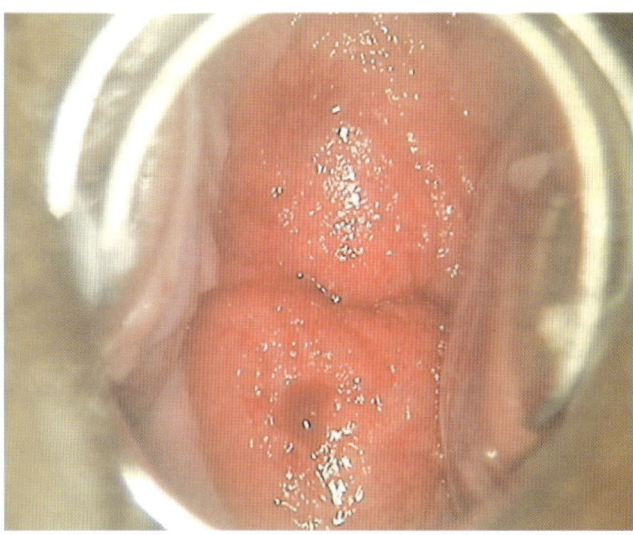

Figure 13-75: Marked eversion of the endocervical columnar epithelium in pregnancy

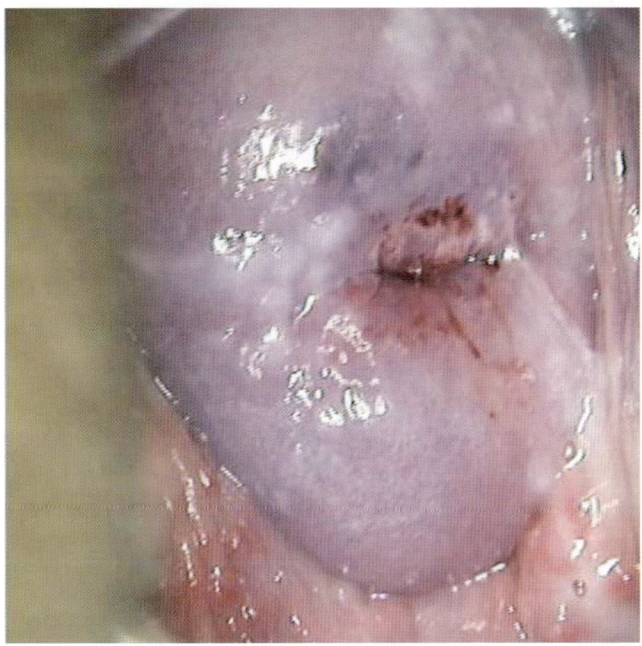

Figure 13-74: Colposcopy picture showing bluish hue of the cervix in pregnancy

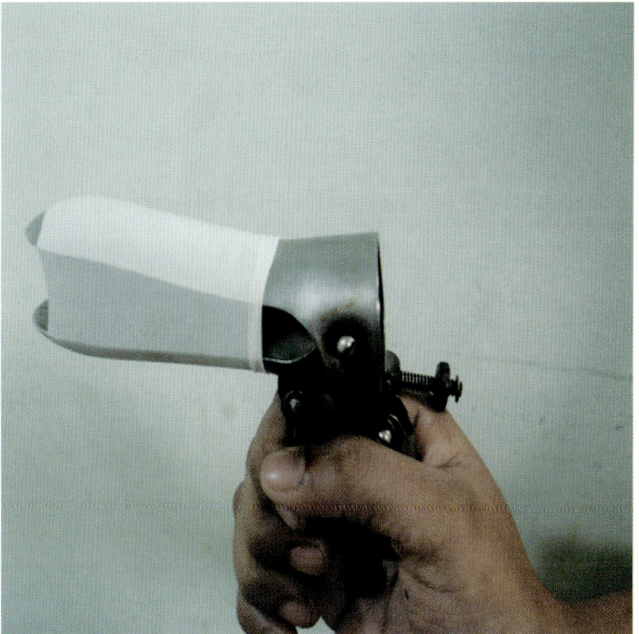

Figure 13-76: Cusco's speculum covered with glove

pregnancy. Because of the decidual changes of pregnancy, the cervix appears polypoidal with raised friable lesions and the vascular pattern may appear atypical. Because of the decidual reaction, the abnormal areas may appear less acetowhite, thereby lesions may be missed.

There may also be difficulty in performing the procedure:
1. Due to laxity of the vaginal wall, it can prolapse through the blades of the speculum and difficulty may be encountered in exposing the cervix.
2. This can be overcome by using a large speculum or lateral vaginal retractors or by covering the speculum by a condom **(Figure 13-76)**.
3. There may be thick tenacious mucus on the cervix which can obscure the view. The mucus can be removed with a sponge holder or the use of acetic acid will dissolve the mucus, or by using cotton-tipped sticks, the mucus can be rotated and kept away from the area of examination.
4. One should be careful in exposing the cervix as there may be heavy bleeding as the cervix is highly vascular.

82   A Practical Approach to Cervical Cancer Screening Techniques

Precautions that are required at the time of colposcopy in pregnancy:
- It is important to reassure the patient that colposcopic assessment of the cervix during pregnancy does not disturb the pregnancy or the fetus.
- The goal of colposcopic examination in pregnant patient with abnormal cytology is to rule out invasive carcinoma; thereby the treatment can be delayed until the postpartum period and any surgical intervention can be postponed.
- If the colposcopist cannot rule out the presence of invasive carcinoma, biopsy should be performed from the area of most significant abnormality and should be kept to a minimum.
- Because of the increased vascularity of the cervix, there may be brisk bleeding after the punch biopsy.
- Colposcopy-directed biopsy can be undertaken in any trimester of pregnancy. Because of the increased risk of bleeding, the number of biopsies should be minimized and, if possible, restricted to only one biopsy from the most affected area.
- Because of the risk of premature rupture of membranes, premature labor and heavy bleeding, endocervical curettage and biopsy should not be done during pregnancy.

Low-grade Intraepithelial Neoplasia

Low-grade intraepithelial neoplasia may have features of condyloma or may show noncondylomatous changes. The acetowhite changes in LSIL are variable. The acetowhite changes exhibited by noncondylomatous lesions are pale, translucent, pale white or pink color. The acetowhite reaction is gradual in onset and more transient in duration than in high-grade lesion. In condylomatous lesions, after acetic acid application, snow-white appearance occurs due to the reflection of the light from the surface keratin.

The noncondylomatous low-grade intraepithelial lesions are flat, the margins are irregular and indistinct, usually described as feathered, flocculated or geographic **(Figures 13-77 to 13-81)**. The LSIL may exhibit punctuation and mosaic pattern. The vessels are fine, of small caliber and with regular distribution. The normal intercapillary distance is maintained (50–250 millimicrons). Atypical vessels are absent.

Condylomatous lesions vary in surface contour from flat lesions to florid exophytic lesions. Some of the lesions may show raised areas with regular projections called asperities. Fine punctuation is a common finding in condylomatous lesions. Each papilla in an exophytic condylomata has a central ascending and descending capillary loop, which is easily seen after acetic acid application. Unlike, exophytic lesions of invasive carcer, condylomata do not show atypical vessels and necrosis **(Figures 13-82 to 13-86)**.

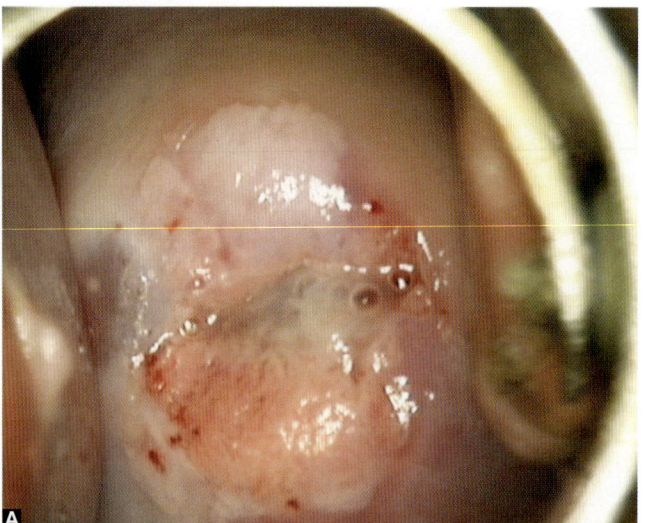
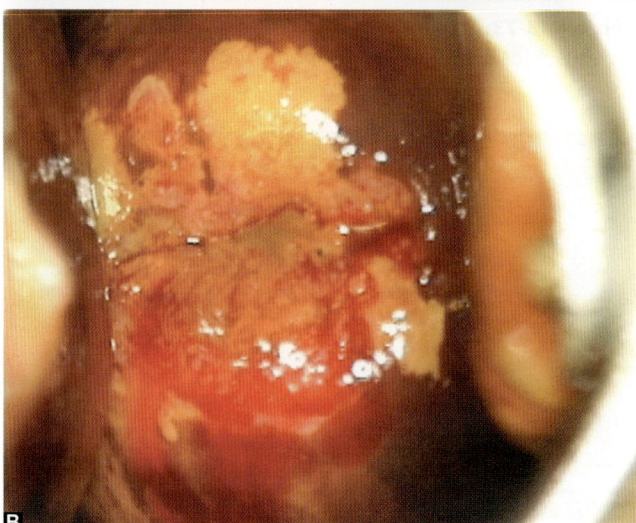

Figures 13-77A and B: Low-grade lesion with faint acetowhite changes and irregular margin, more marked in the anterior lip of the cervix

Difficulties in Interpreting Low-grade Lesions

- The physiological changes of immature metaplasia and reparative changes following treatment with cryotherapy or loop excision may be confused with low-grade lesions. The above conditions also exhibit faint translucent acetowhite changes, irregular margin, punctuation and mosaics.
- In postmenopausal women, due to the thinning of the squamous epithelium and the presence of only basal and parabasal layer, there may be blunting of acetowhite changes and surface contour; therefore, a high-grade lesion may be underestimated as a low-grade lesion.
- In pregnancy the interpretation of low grade lesion is difficult.

Interpretations of Colposcopy Findings

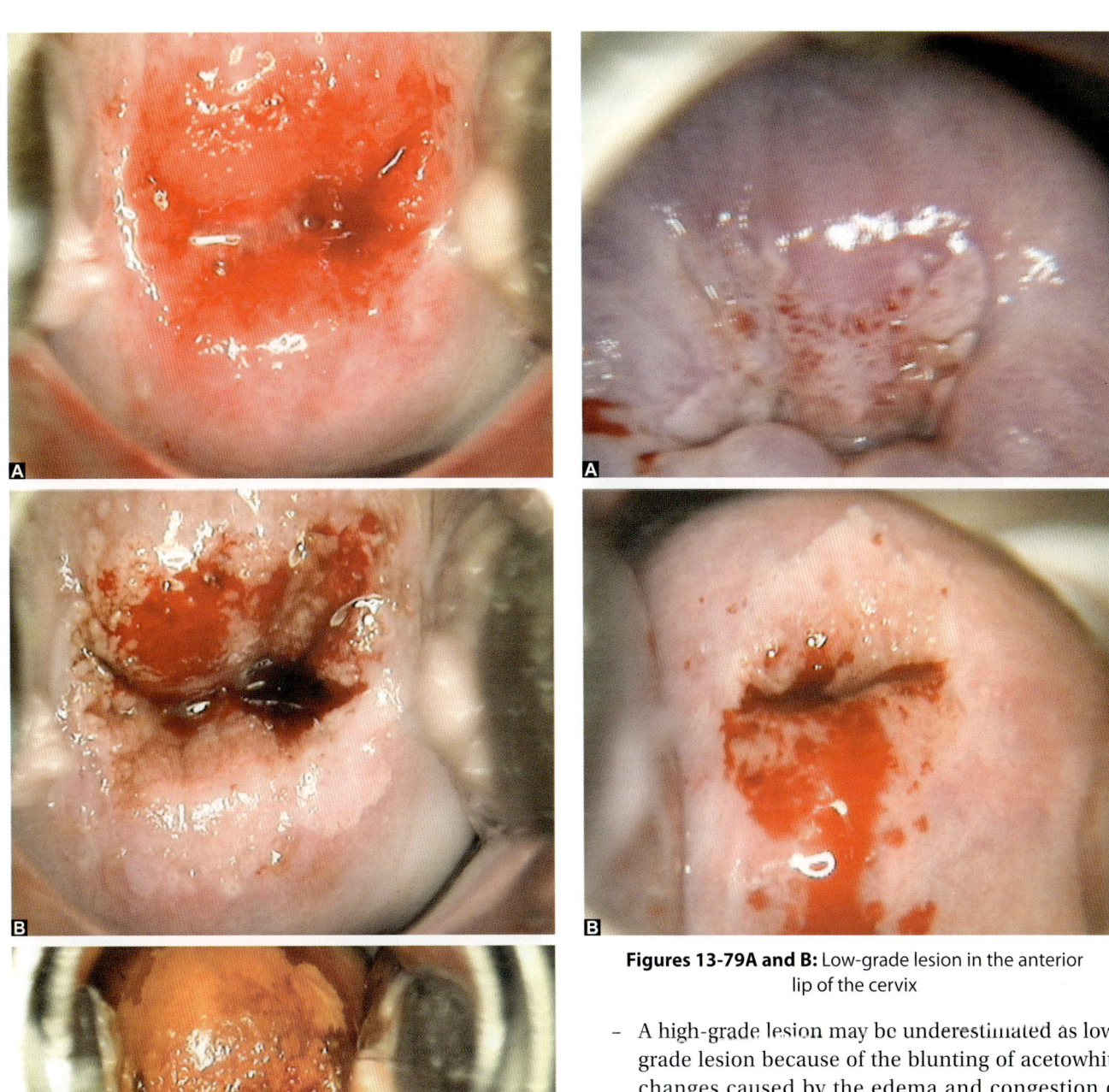

Figures 13-78A to C: A large low-grade lesion with irregular margin and faint acetowhite changes. The lesion is avascular

Figures 13-79A and B: Low-grade lesion in the anterior lip of the cervix

- A high-grade lesion may be underestimated as low-grade lesion because of the blunting of acetowhite changes caused by the edema and congestion of pregnancy
- The metaplastic changes caused by the eversion of the endocervical canal in pregnancy may be overestimated as a low-grade lesion.

Colposcopy Findings in High-Grade Lesions (Figures 13-87 to 13-90)

High-grade lesions may be found anywhere in the TZ, but more often seen closer to the SCJ. A high-grade lesion may be seen within a large low-grade lesion, with a clear line of demarcation. This is called internal margin, and is a reliable

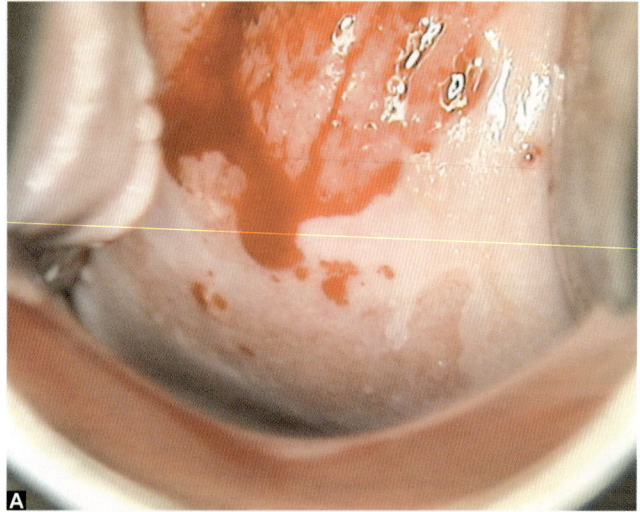

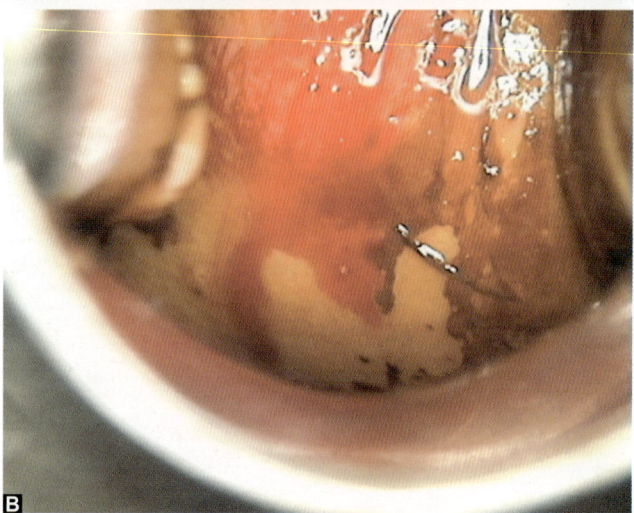

Figures 13-80A and B: Faint acetowhite epithelium and geographic border in a low-grade lesion

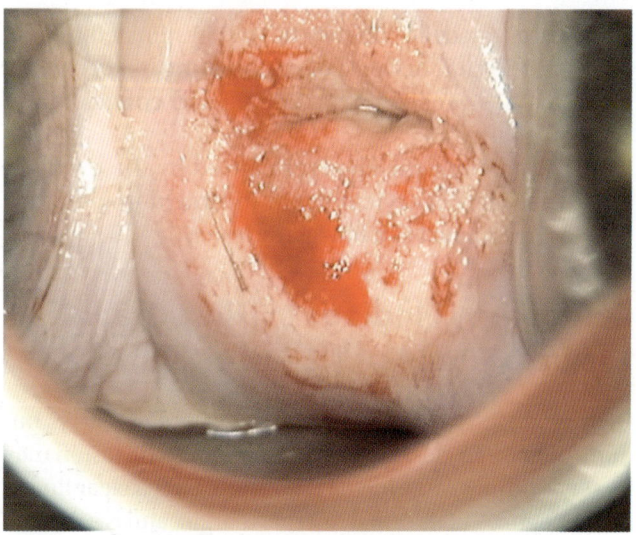

Figure 13-81: A low-grade lesion showing a large area of acetowhite epithelium with fine punctation at 5 o'clock position

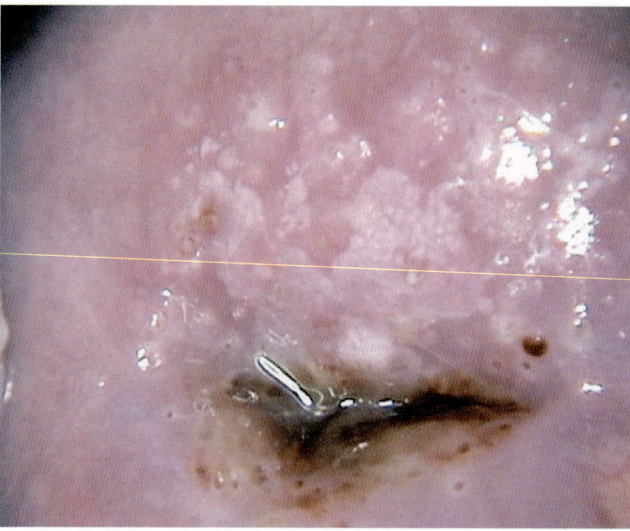

Figure 13-82: Diffusely scattered acetowhite lesions indicating HPV infection. There is a dense acetowhite lesion with internal margin at 12 o'clock position indicating the presence of a high-grade lesion

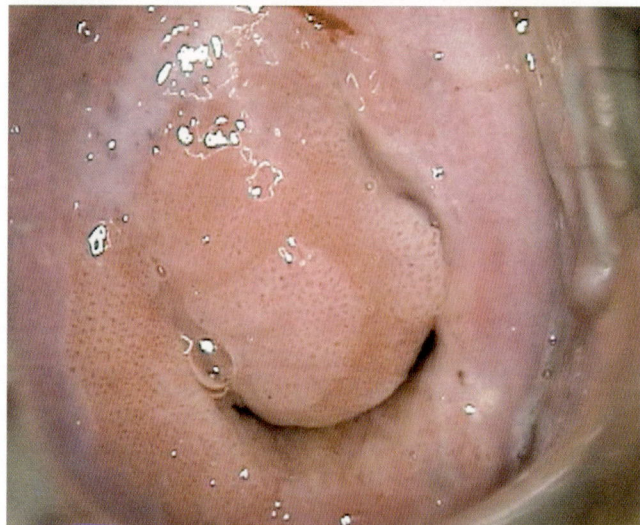

Figure 13-83: Large exophytic condyloma at the external os of cervix. The posterior lip of the cervix shows coarse punctation

sign of high-grade cervical disease. High-grade lesions often show raised surface contour with peeling and rolled edges. This peeling is due to inability of the cells to adhere to one another due to the loss of desmosomes. The lesions have straight, sharp and very distinctive peripheral margins. Because of this distinctive feature, the abnormal area can be clearly demarcated from the normal area.

The acetowhite changes may be denser than the low-grade lesions. They are dull and not shiny due to the increased nuclear content and less reflection of light. The acetowhite changes appear quick and remain for a longer time.

Interpretations of Colposcopy Findings 85

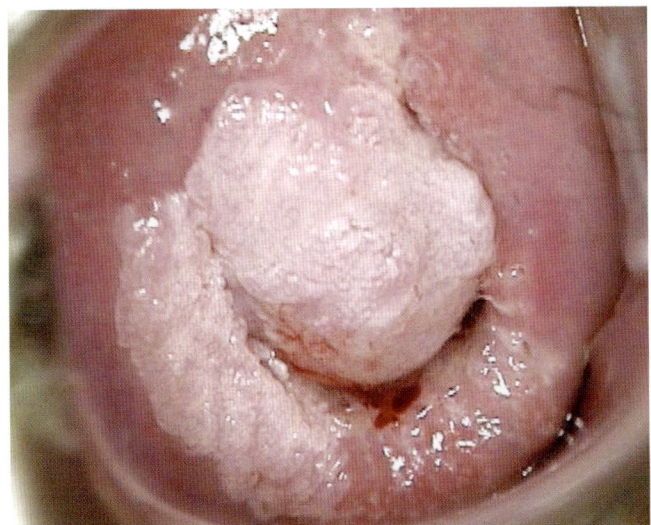

Figure 13-84: A condylomatous lesion which appears snow-white after acetic acid application

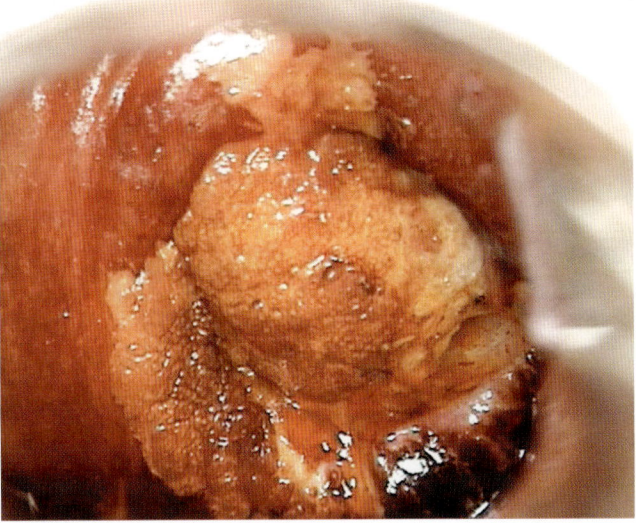

Figure 13-85: Condylomatous lesion which is iodine negative

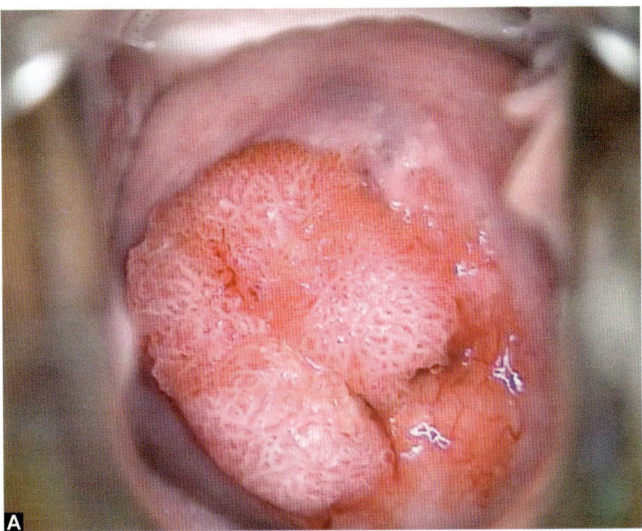

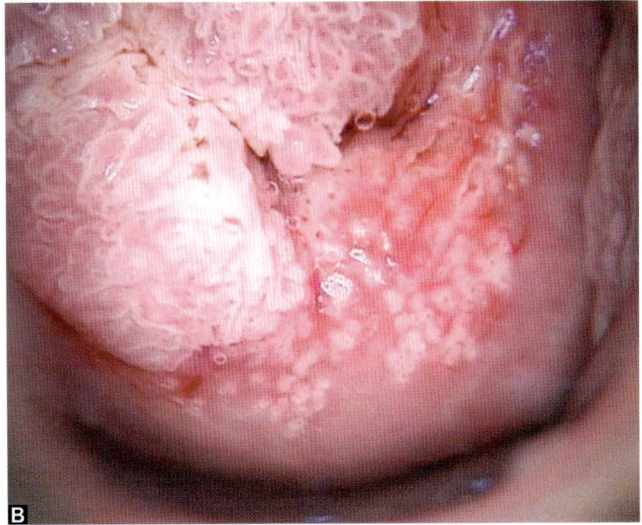

Figures 13-86A and B: A large exophytic condyloma at the external os. A. The TZ between 3 and 7 o'clock positions shows atypical vessels; B. Scattered acetowhite areas in the TZ

On inspection through a green filter, one can find abnormal vascular pattern with coarse punctuation and/ or mosaics. In some cases, these vascular changes may not be evident after application of 3% to 5% acetic acid. This is due to the constriction of the narrow vessels caused by the intense swelling of the dysplastic epithelium. Therefore, in some cases, absence of vessels may be noted. Therefore, the presence or absence of a vascular pattern is not diagnostic of either a high-grade lesion or a low-grade lesion. As the vascular dilatation becomes more, it resists the vasoconstrictive effect of the dysplastic epithelium; thus mosaics and punctation will be evident after acetic acid application. As the vascularity is increased, the inter-vascular distance increases, the vessels get dilated, and they begin to course horizontally across the surface; thus, the abnormal vascular pattern becomes atypical.

In high-grade lesions, the surface epithelium detaches very easily. Therefore, care must be taken at colposcopy and cotton-tipped applicator should be used very gently if manipulation is required. Adequate number of biopsies should be taken from the most abnormal areas. Colposcopically, the epithelial detachment appears as rolled or peeling edges.

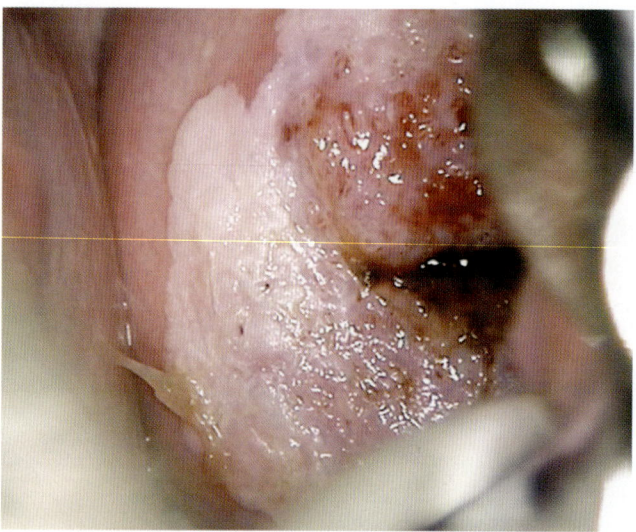

Figure 13-87: A high-grade lesion with raised dense acetowhite epithelium. High-grade lesions

Colposcopy in Invasive Cancer (Figures 13-91 and 13-92)

The abnormal colposcopy findings indicative of invasive cervical carcinomas are similar to the colposcopy findings seen in preinvasive cancers, such as acetowhite epithelium, mosaics, punctation and atypical vessels. It is believed that the pathognomonic of invasive cancer is the presence of atypical vessels, which are more prominent as the depth of invasion increases. The vessels are 2 to 10 times wider than the normal capillaries, irregular in width, shape and course. Other features which are commonly seen are areas of necrosis, which appear yellow, ulceration and exophytic mass.

Colposcopy Findings in Adenocarcinoma In Situ and Adenocarcinoma

Because of the endocervical location and glandular architecture, the neoplastic glands are difficult to locate and are often buried under the surface. Therefore, in ACIS and adenocarcinoma, the surface contour changes are very minimal. Glandular lesions can be easily missed both by exfoliate cytology and at colposcopy. Glandular lesions are often associated with squamous lesions. At exfoliative cytology, the abnormal squamous cells are easily identified; therefore, they will be reported as squamous cell abnormality. This report can easily influence the Colposcopist to look for squamous abnormality, thus missing the endocervical lesion.

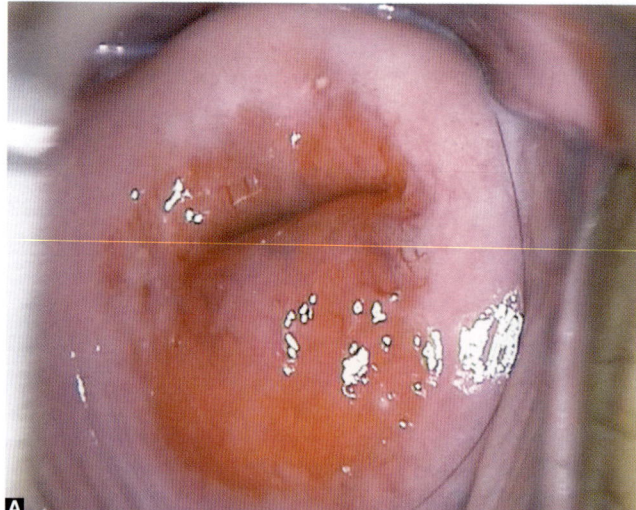
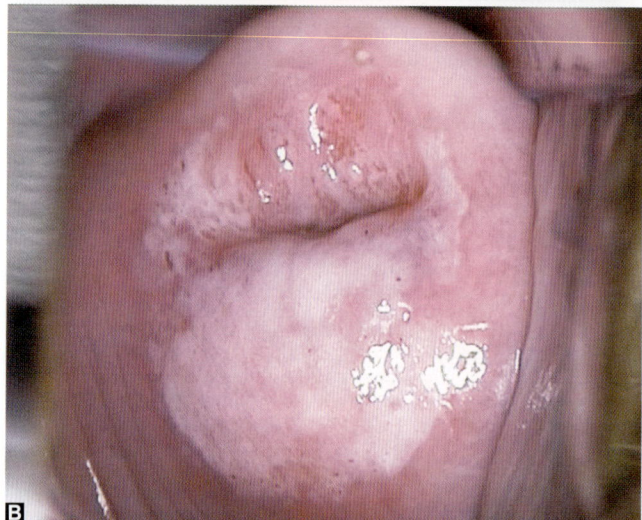
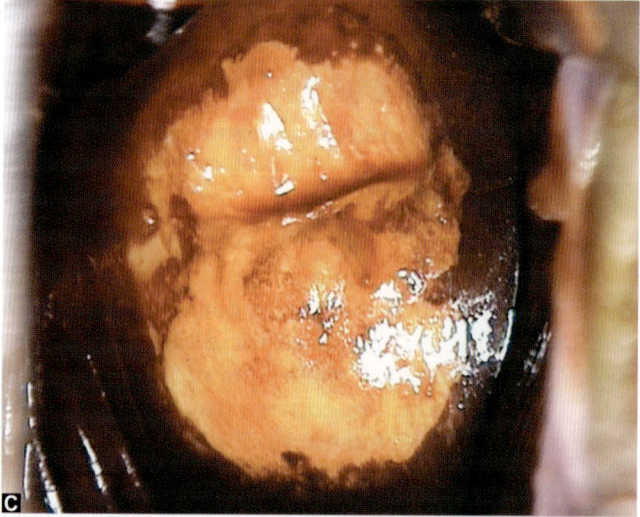

Figures 13-88A to C: A large dense acetowhite lesion on the posterior lip of the cervix. The lesion has a clear demarcation and is avascular indicating high-grade lesion. The anterior lip of the cervix shows a low-grade lesion with fine punctation. The lesion is iodine negative

Interpretations of Colposcopy Findings

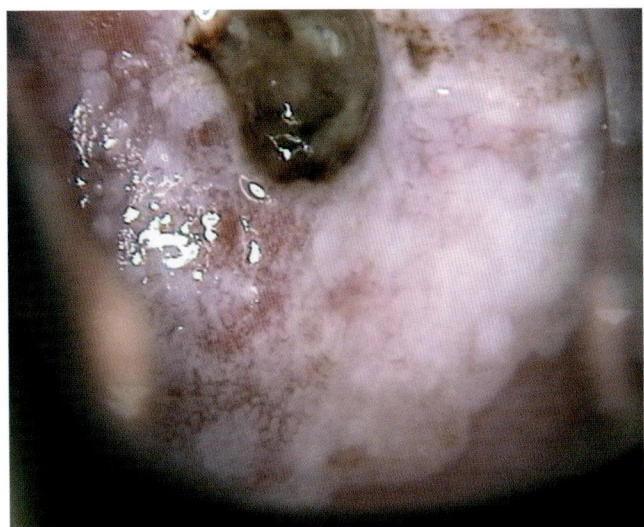

Figure 13-89: A high-grade lesion having dense acetowhite changes, coarse mosaics and clear margin

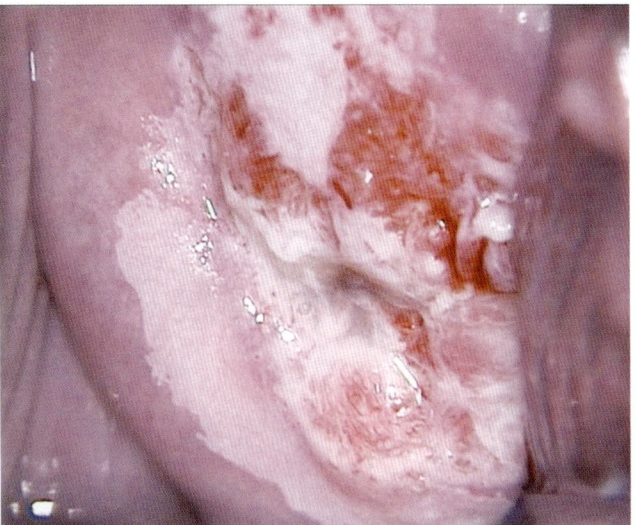

Figure 13-91: A lesion having dense acetowhite changes, coarse mosaics and atypical vessels in the anterior and posterior lips. Biopsy confirmed the presence of invasive carcinoma

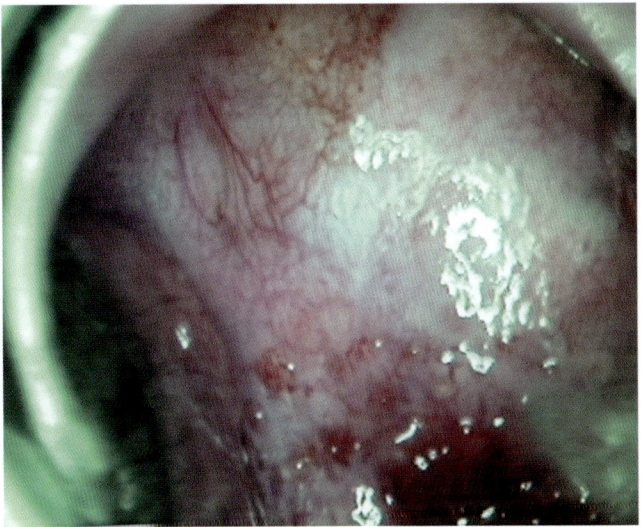

Figure 13-90: A High-grade lesion. The mosaics get accentuated when seen through the green filter

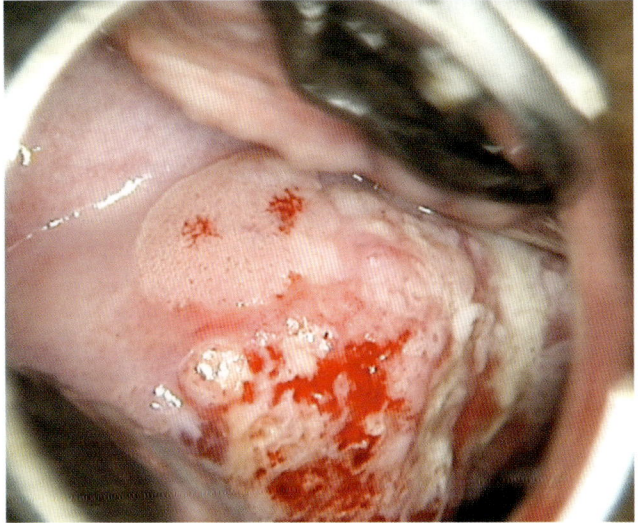

Figure 13-92: A lesion having raised acetowhite areas and coarse punctation and mosaics. Part of the lesion shows ulceration with peeling edges. Findings are consistent with invasive carcinoma

At colposcopy, glandular lesion should be suspected in the presence of the following findings **(Figures 13-93A and B)**.
- The presence of acetowhite papillary epithelium at the glandular location or close to the TZ (unlike the squamous lesions, glandular lesions are not contiguous with SCJ). The papillary appearance is due to the presence of fused villi
- The presence of patchy, raised dense acetowhite areas over the columnar epithelium
- The presence of large 'gland' like openings
- The presence of epithelial budding—ACIS can proliferate like 'cactus' budding
- Atypical blood vessels may present with waste-thread, tendril, root-like and character-writing patterns
- Punctation, mosaics and corkscrew vessels, which are typical of squamous lesions, are not seen in glandular lesions
- Presence of two or more squamous lesions separated by a gland-like epithelium is highly suggestive of a glandular lesion

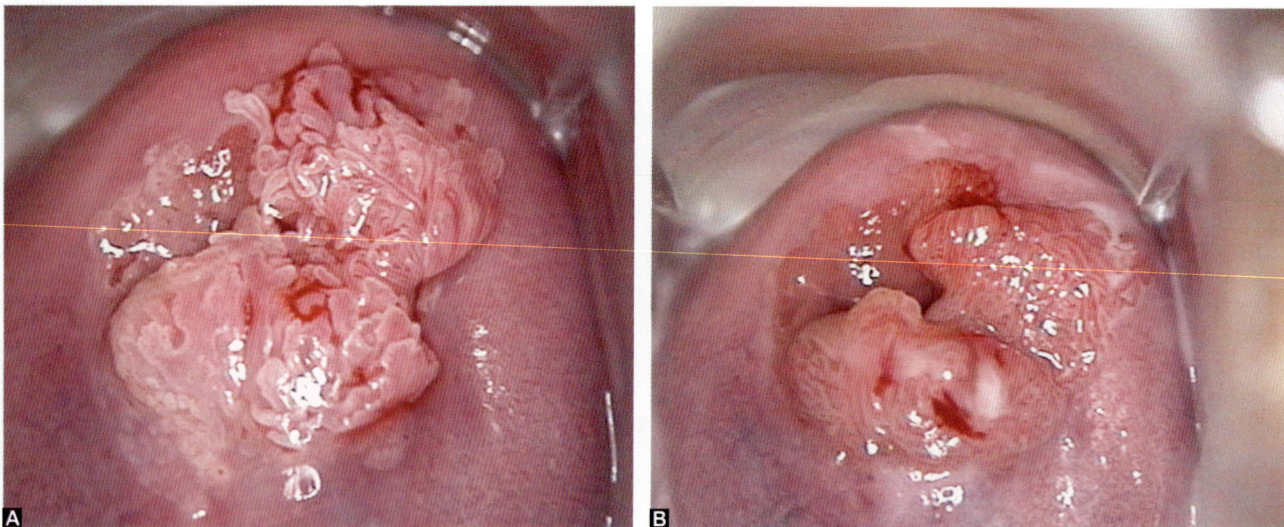

Figures 13-93A and B: Cactus-like proliferation of glandular epithelium with acetowhite lesions over the posterior lip

- ACIS can be multifocal with 'skip' lesions.
- RCI cannot be used for reporting glandular lesions

Presence of acetowhite papillary epithelium and patchy red and white areas is also there in immature metaplasia and condylomas.

Nearly 50% of ACIS are associated with squamous lesions.

Squamous cell carcinomas are seen in 4–5% of mixed disease.

Irrespitive of the age, fertility status and lesion location, diagnostic excision biopsy should be done when ACIS was found on biopsy or when suspected cytologically or colposcopically, but not proven by histopathology.

Chapter 14

Visual Inspection Methods (VIA and VILI)

The major problems in organizing cytological screening in developing countries are as follows:
1. Financial constraints and difficulties in organizing cervical screening programs in countries with vast population
2. Lack of clinical expertise, trained physicians, nurses and technicians to carry out cytological screening
3. Inability to maintain the quality in interpreting Pap smear samples
4. Confirmatory testing with colposcopy and biopsy is not available in all the centers
5. Limited availability of treatment facilities
6. Difficulties in the follow-up of patients.

Because of the above challenges in implementing high-quality Pap smear services in the developing countries, the Alliance for Cervical Cancer Prevention (ACCP) has studied alternative screening methods, namely visual screening and HPV testing.

Visual Screening Techniques

1. Visual inspection with acetic acid (VIA)
2. Visual inspection with acetic acid under low magnification (VIAM)
3. Visual inspection with Lugol's iodine (VILI)

Advantages of Visual Screening

1. It is simple, low-cost and minimal infrastructure is required. Therefore, it is useful in low-resource settings
2. After adequate training and under supervision, even nonmedical personnel, such as ANMS/VHNS can perform the procedure
3. As the result of the test is available immediately, during the same visit either referral or treatment can be offered.

The visual approaches to cervical cancer screening by VIA, VILI, VIAM depend upon the color changes imparted by the chemicals, namely acetic acid and Lugol's iodine on the cervix. These color changes are observed with naked eye or under low magnification.

Disadvantages of Visual Screening

1. Healthcare workers should be trained adequately to recognize subtle changes in the cervix to diagnose abnormal areas. This would be a major challenge, and intense training and monitoring are required.
2. Number of physiological changes in the cervix, such as metaplasia can impart color changes with acetic and Lugol's iodine. Therefore, healthy women may be diagnosed with abnormal cell changes and this false positive result can be the cause of overtreatment, as well as women would be subjected to psychological stress.
3. In postmenopausal women, the TZ recedes into the endocervical canal; therefore, it is difficult to diagnose abnormalities within the endocervix. External cervical os may appear apparently healthy, but a lesion may lie within the cervical canal, which can be easily missed.
4. Some of the developing countries practice single visit approach, wherein cryotherapy is offered once VIA/VILI is positive. Here the diagnosis cannot be proved by histology. This can result in undertreatment of severe grades of CIN lesions.

Other Issues Related to Visual Screening

1. What is the screening frequency?
2. What should be the treatment once the diagnosis is made?
3. When is the follow-up required?

Inspite of the above shortcomings, IARC recommends (IARC 2005) that in very low resource settings, VIA may be a viable alternative to cytology.[61]

VISUAL INSPECTION WITH ACETIC ACID (VIA)

Basis of VIA

Acetic acid application to the cervix results in precipitation and coagulation of nuclear proteins of the cells. It also causes swelling and dehydration of the epithelial tissue. This coagulation by acetic acid imparts a white appearance to the cells—the 'acetowhite change'. This acetowhite appearance is transient and reversible.

Precancer cells have more nuclear protein and absent or minimal glycogen. Depending upon the nuclear activity and nuclear protein content, the intensity of acetowhite changes can vary from shiny, faint acetowhite changes, to cloudy dull-oyster white appearance to very dense opaque-acetowhiteness.

During the procedure, one should also observe the rapidity of appearance and the disappearance of acetowhite changes to the cervix.

EFFECT OF ACETIC ACID ON VARIOUS TISSUES

Effect of Acetic Acid on Squamous Epithelium

In the squamous epithelium, the deeper layers, namely basal and parabasal cells contain more nuclear protein as the size of the nucleus is large. The superficial and intermediate layers contain less nuclear material.

When acetic acid (AA) is applied to the normal squamous epithelium, the AA does not penetrate deep enough to coagulate the nuclear protein on basal and parabasal cells. Therefore, the precipitation from the superficial layers is not sufficient enough to obscure the color of the underlying stroma. Therefore, the squamous epithelium maintains the normal pale pink appearance.

Effect of Acetic Acid on Columnar Epithelium

When AA is applied to the columnar epithelium due to the mucus content of the columnar cells, there is transient faint acetowhiteness which disappears quickly and the villi pattern will be clearly visible.

Effect of Acetic Acid on Other Epithelia

In immature squamous metaplasia and healing and regenerating epithelium, due to active division of cells, the nuclear content of the cells is increased.

The nuclear content of the cells is also increased in CIN lesions due to high number of undifferentiated cells in the epithelium. Condylomas and leukoplakic lesions (hyperkeratinization) also contain more nuclear protein.

Therefore, CIN, invasive lesions, condylomas leukoplakic areas, immature squamous metaplasia and regenerating epithelium, all will turn white with acetic acid application.

However, the characteristic features such as intensity and duration of whiteness, the borders of lesions as well as the proximity to the TZ will delineate, whether the lesion is normal or abnormal.

Intensity and Duration of Whiteness

Inflammatory and healing lesions show shiny, faint and very transient acetowhite changes. Metaplastic lesions produce pale, thin and translucent whiteness.

Leukoplakia and condylomas show intense greying white changes.

Abnormal areas with CIN and invasive carcinoma show dense opaque acetowhiteness or dull oyster-white appearance. In these cases, acetowhiteness appears rapidly and lasts for three to five minutes.

Borders of the Lesion

In CIN lesions, the demarcation between the normal and abnormal will be sharp and distinct and the abnormal acetowhite area will have a regular margin.

In inflammation and metaplastic areas, the demarcation is diffuse; the area is flat with irregular margin. Angular and finger-like acetowhite projection can be seen arising from the SCJ.

Location of the Lesion

Abnormal areas are seen close to or arising from the SCJ in the TZ or close to the ectocervix, if the SCJ is not visible.

Inflammation and healing lesions are not restricted to TZ, distributed widely in the cervix.

Satellite lesions can be seen away from the SCJ. Condylomatous lesions can be seen away from the TZ. In metaplastic lesions, angular, finger-like projection from the SCJ (geographical lesions) and satellite lesions away from the SCJ are seen.

Visual Inspection with Lugol's Iodine (VILI)

Basis of VILI

Normal tissues will have adequate glycogen content. When iodine solution is applied to a normal tissue, a mahogany brown color appears.

Epithelium that contains little or no glycogen does not take up the stain. Columnar epithelium, metaplastic epithelium and atypical cells lack glycogen. Therefore, do not take up iodine.

Procedure of VIA and VILI

Instruments and Material Required

1. Examination table with stirrups
2. Good light source
3. Cusco's speculum of varying sizes
4. Gloves
5. Cotton swabs
6. Ring forceps
7. Cups for chemicals
8. 5% acetic acid with Lugol's iodine
9. Magnavision, if magnification is used (**Figure 14-1**). With this simple instrument, magnification can be achieved four times.

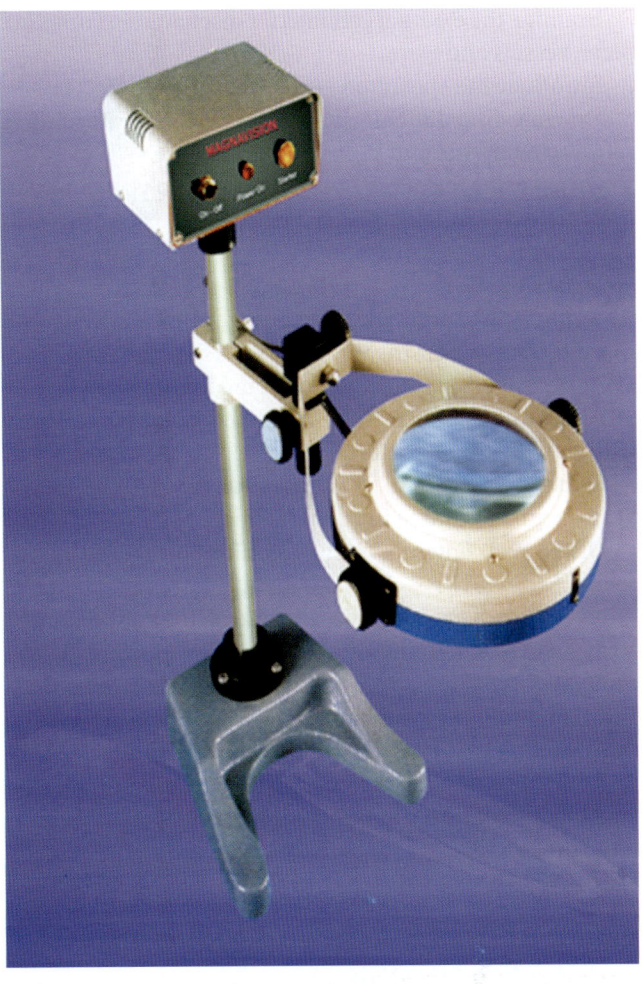

Figure 14-1: Magnavision

> **INFORMED CONSENT FOR VIA AND VILI**
>
> I, Mrs X, give my consent for the procedure of Vinegar test (VIA)/Iodine test (VILI). The healthcare personnel have explained to me the need for cervical cancer screening. I have been explained that VIA and VILI are the tests used for the early detection of precancerous changes that occur in the neck of the womb (cervix).
>
> I have been explained that the cervix and the vagina will be washed with 5% acetic acid/iodine solution to look for abnormal changes on the cervix. I have been told that if there are abnormal changes, I will need further examination of the cervix under magnification with an instrument called colposcope, if necessary tissue sample may be taken from the cervix (biopsy) before the treatment is offered.
>
> I have been told that the procedure does not required anesthesia, and the use of vinegar may cause some irritation which is transient.
>
> I have been explained that by the above tests, if abnormalities are detected on the cervix, the diseased portion of the cervix may be removed or destroyed by a minor surgery.

Technique of VIA and VILI

Procedure explained:
    Informed consent obtained
    Relevant history taken
    Ask the patient to empty the bladder
    Position the patient

Examine the external genitalia for discharge, excoriation, ulcer, vessels and warts

Introduce the speculum and expose the cervix

One may find difficulty in exposing the cervix in acutely retroverted uterus and in cases of previous CS

On exposing the cervix, look for ectopy, polyp, nabothian cyst, condyloma, leukoplakia, cervicitis, erosion, vaginitis and growth

Locate the SCJ

Apply acetic acid, allow acetic acid to react for one minute, then report the findings

Apply Lugol's Iodine and report the findings.

Also look for abnormal changes in the vagina while slowly withdrawing the speculum

Once the examination is complete remove the excess acetic acid and Iodine from the vagina.

Disposal of contaminants and sterilization of used instruments:

After the procedure is over, dispose off the contaminated swabs and gauze in the respective plastic buckets. Before removing the gloves, rinse the hand with containing 0.5% chlorine solution. Decontamination can be done by soaking the gloves in 0.5% chlorine solution for 10 minutes.

Nondisposable instruments are first decontaminated by soaking in chlorine solution for 10 minutes, then washed and autoclaved.

Effect of Acetic Acid and Iodine on Cervical Epithelium

3–5% Acetic Acid Application

Before acetic acid application, the normal translucent epithelium reflects the underlying vascular connective tissue

Squamous epithelium appears pale pink due to multiple layers of cells

Columnar epithelium appears bright red due to the single-layer cell

When acetic acid is applied, it coagulates the cellular protein, especially the cytokeratin. This biochemical change is seen through the colposcope as a whitening or opaqueness occurring within the visible epithelium

This change is transient and reversible

Normal epithelium has minimal amount of protein and large amounts of glycogen

Therefore, when normal squamous epithelium is washed with acetic acid, it remains unchanged, retaining the translucent pink color

The columnar epithelium because of the mucus content can become transiently white; however, the villi pattern will show the presence of columnar epithelium

In atypical epithelium, there is protein in cell membrane, and increase in nuclear protein and very little glycogen So, the squamous epithelium becomes progressively opaque, a dull appearance that masks the reflection of the underlying connective tissue. In major-grade lesions, the opacity of the lesion becomes whiter.

Lugol's Iodine Application—Schiller's Test

Normal tissues will have adequate glycogen content

When iodine solution is applied to a normal tissue, a mahogany brown color appears

Epithelium, that contains little or no glycogen, does not take up the stain.

Reporting the Results of VIA

After application of acetic acid, the outcome is reported as either VIA negative (–) or VIA positive (+).

VIA NEGATIVE

If any of the following observations are made, the screening is reported as negative:

1. No acetowhite lesion observed on the cervix
2. Polyps protruding from the cervix with bluish white acetowhite areas
3. Button-like acetowhite areas distributed over the TZ—indicating nabothian cysts
4. Transient faint acetowhite changes seen in columnar epithelium
5. Shiny, faint cloudy white, bluish white patchy lesion with irregular margin, blending with the rest of the cervix, indicating metaplastic changes
6. Faint line like ill-defined acetowhiteness at SCJ
7. Angular, irregular, digitating acetowhite lesion, geographical lesion from the SCJ or satellite lesion, which is away from the SCJ indicating metaplasia **(Figure 14-2)**
8. Diffuse transient acetowhiteness scattered over the entire cervix indicating infection.

VIA POSITIVE

The test is reported positive in the presence of the following findings:

1. Distinct, well-defined dense opaque or dull oyster white acetowhite areas close to or abutting the SCJ in the TZ or close to the external os if the SCJ is not visualized **(Figure 14-3)**
2. Strikingly dense acetowhite areas in the columnar epithelium
3. Condyloma and leukoplakia close to the SCJ turning intensely white after application of acetic acid.

Visual Inspection Methods (VIA and VILI)

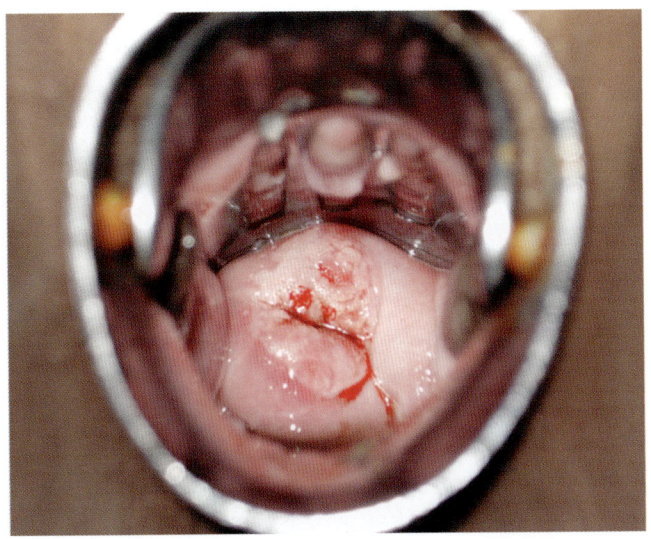

Figure 14-2: Irregular, digitating, faint acetowhite areas around the SCJ after applying acetic acid to the cervix

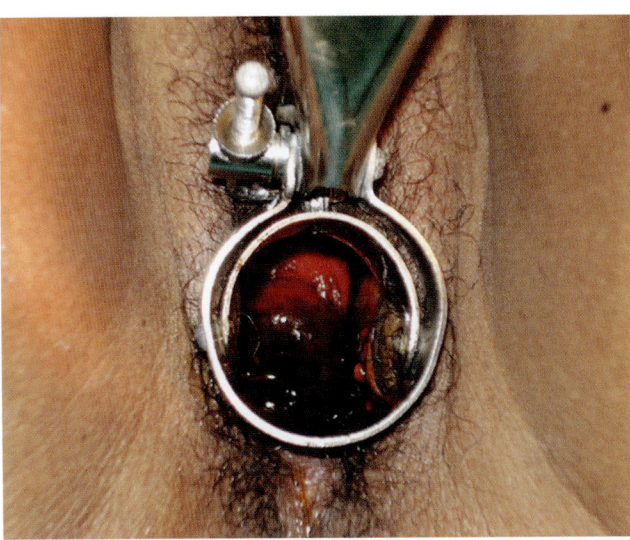

Figure 14-4: Normal cervix which stains mahogany brown/black after Lugol's iodine application

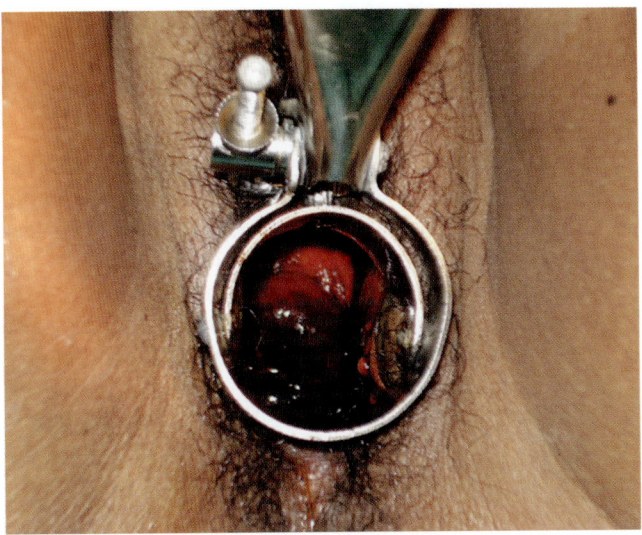

Figure 14-3: Raised, very distinct, dense acetowhite lesion around the external os, more prominent in the anterior lip of the cervix

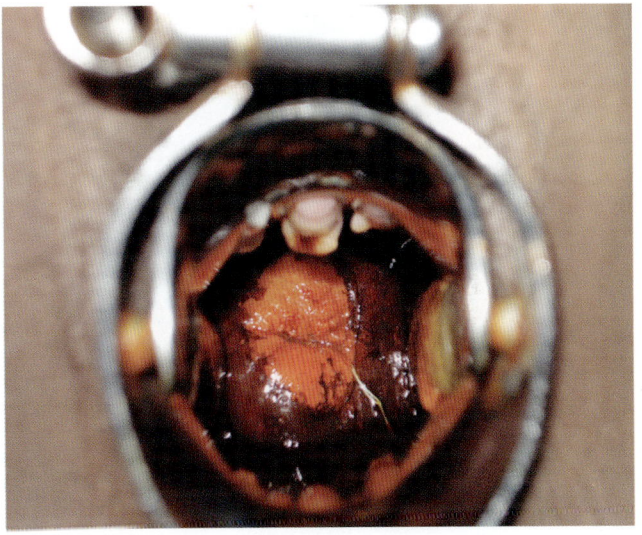

Figure 14-5: Yellow noniodine-staining areas with irregular margins

Outcome of VILI

VILI is reported as either positive or negative
  VILI negative (−) **(Figures 14-4 to 14-7)**
  The squamous epithelium of normal cervix turns mahogany brown or black due to the good glycogen content. Columnar epithelium does not change color (Columnar epithelium lacks glycogen)
  Polyps showing absent or areas of partial iodine uptake
  Patchy noniodine-stained areas distributed widely on the cervix and vagina (Leopard skin appearance). Seen commonly in *Trichomonas vaginalis* infection
  Dotted nonstained areas on the squamous epithelium away from the SCJ (Pepper-like lesions). Seen in infection, inflammation and ulceration of the cervix
  Thin, yellow, noniodine uptake areas with angular or digitating margins away from the SCJ-Geographical areas seen in metaplasia
  Thin yellow noniodine-staining areas away from the SCJ and satellite lesions seen in metaplasia

94 A Practical Approach to Cervical Cancer Screening Techniques

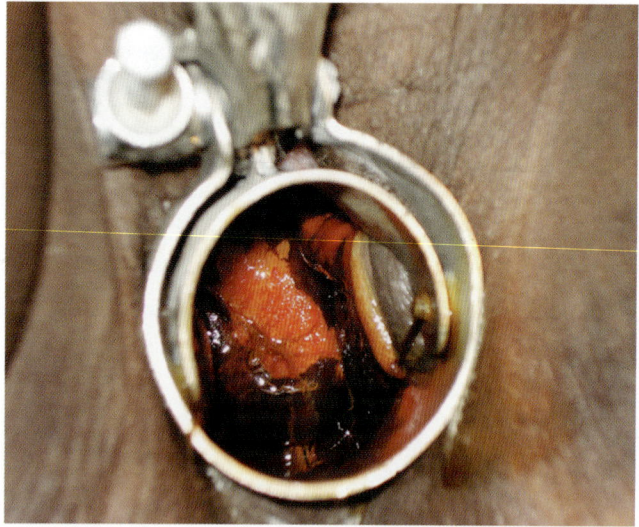

Figure 14-6: Yellow, noniodine-staining area with satellite lesion detached from the SCJ

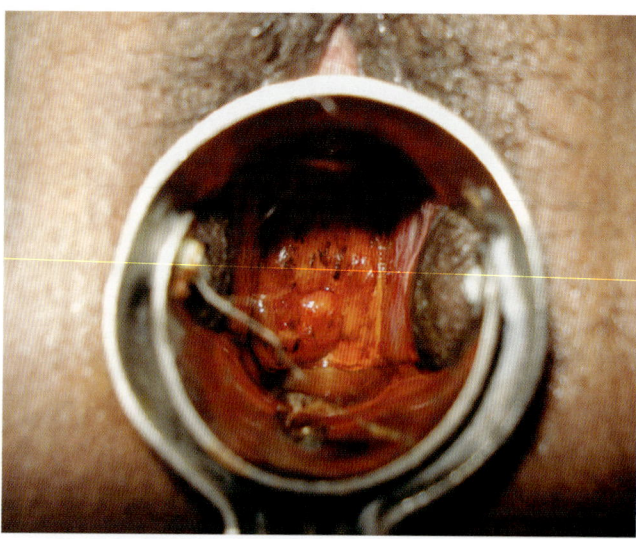

Figure 14-8: Yellow iodine non-uptake areas with clear margin

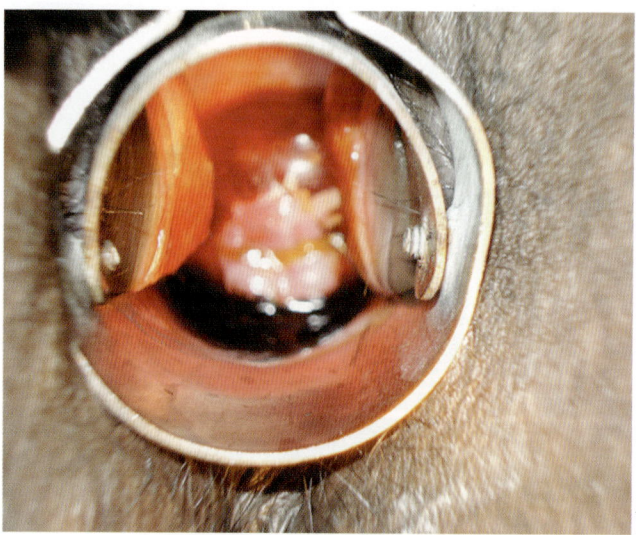

Figure 14-7: Iodine negative area with irregular digitating margin. The columnar epithelium does not take up iodine

VILI Positive (Figure 14-8)

Dense thick, bright, mustard yellow or saffron-yellow iodine nonuptake areas seen in TZ, close to the SCJ or abutting from the SCJ or close to the cervix if the SCJ is not visible.

Invasive Cancer

Frank, nodular, irregular, ulceroproliferative growth visible on the cervix, which turns densely yellow on application if iodine is there on the cervix. It may involve all quadrants of cervix and extend into the cervical canal.

Leukoplakic lesions: These appear as white raised keratinized areas and these do not stain with iodine.

Condylomas: Do not stain with iodine.

Documentation of results (Figure 14-9):
  Whether VIA positive or negative or invasive carcinoma?
  Whether VILI positive or negative or invasive carcinoma?
  Whether the acetowhite lesion/iodine negative area extends into the endocervical canal?
  Document the extent of the lesion in quadrants
  Draw the squamocolumnar junction in dotted line and acetowhite and iodine negative areas are represented as a continuous line.
  Whether biopsy has been taken? If yes, enclose the report.

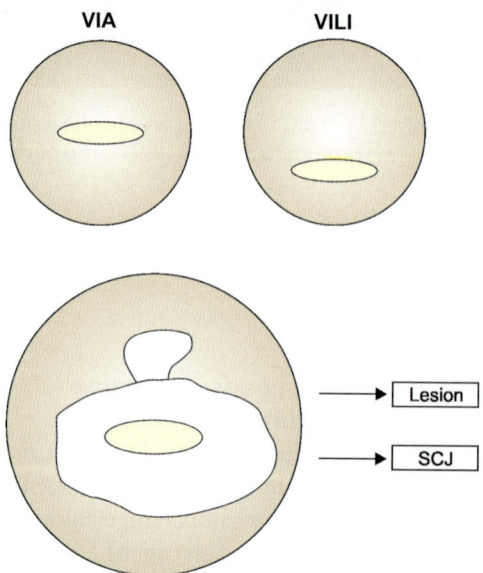

Figure 14-9: Documentation of results

Table 14-1: Result of VIA in various cervical conditions

S.no	Condition	Intensity of acetowhiteness	Borders	Location
1.	Inflammation/Reparative changes	Shiny, faint, transient	Demarcation diffuse, irregular margin	Not restricted to T2, distributed widely on the cervix
2.	Metaplasia	Pale, thin, translucent whiteness	Demarcation diffuse, irregular margin, angular, finger-like acetowhite projections from SCJ	Angular acetowhite lesions extending from SCJ (Geographical lesion). Satellite lesions away from the SCJ
3.	Leukoplakia	White lesion before applying acetic acid		
4.	Condylomata	Intense grey white lesions	Regular margin sharp demarcation from normal epithelium, diffuse lesions	Seen near as well as away from TZ. Multiple exophytic lesions in cervix and vagina.
5.	CIN lesions	Dense opaque/dull oyster white appearance. Acetowhiteness appears rapidly and lasts for a longer time	Regular margins, sharp and distinct borders	Seen close to or arising from the SCJ in the TZ or close to the ectocervix if the SCJ is not visible.
6.	Invasive carcinoma	Dense acetowhite areas with irregular surface	Raised and rolled out margins with peeling edges	Ulceroproliferative growth at the external os.

Treatment

If test result was negative, give instructions to the woman as to when to come for the follow-up.

If test result was positive,
  Whether immediate treatment was given?
  Whether referred for colposcopy?
  What was the post-treatment follow-up?

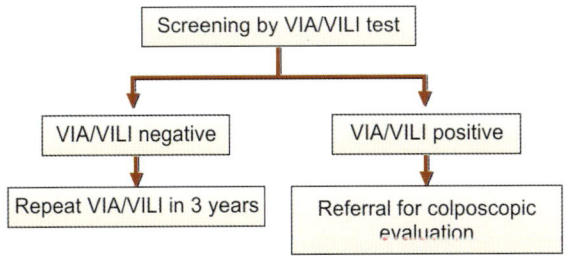

Figure 14-10: Protocol to be followed after VIA/VILI test result

Efficacy of VIA and VILI

Various studies have looked into the accuracy of visual screening techniques for cervical neoplasia.

In a cross-sectional study by Sankaranarayanan et al. (2003) in Kerala, India, the test results of VIA, VILI and conventional cytology were studied in 4444 women. Their study indicated that VIA and VILI are suitable alternate screening tests to cytology for detecting cervical neoplasia in low-resource setting.[62]

In order to assess the cost-effectiveness of various screening methods, a cluster randomized trial was conducted on 131,178 women in rural India. It was found that screening with VIA was the least expensive option, but it also detected fewer cases of CIN 2/3 than other methods. Cytology was more effective at detecting cases than VIA but it was also more expensive. The study also indicated that HPV may not be a cost-effective screening strategy.[63]

A study by IARC Multicentric Study Group on cervical cancer early detection showed that the efficacy of VIA for the detection of HSIL was 76.8% sensitive (95% CI 74.2–79.4%), 85.5% specific (95% CI 85.2%-85.8%) with a positive predictive value of 9.4% and a negative predictive value of 99.5%). The results of VIA were compared with the results of Lugol's Iodine (VILI) and it was found that the sensitivity of VILI was significantly higher than VIA, in detecting HSIL but the specificity remained same. The study recommended that VILI appears to be a more accurate visual test for use in screening in low-resource settings.[64]

Chapter 15

Cell Cycle Markers

There has been recent interest and research in identifying cell cycle markers by means of immunocytochemistry.

In cervical carcinogenesis, there is an integration of high-risk HPV DNA into the host cell genomes. This results in elevated expression of the E6 and E7 proteins, which in turn, interact with the cell cycle regulatory genes.

Major regulatory events leading to cell proliferation and differentiation occur within the G_1 phase of the cell cycle and the cell cycle is governed by a family of cyclins, namely cyclin-dependent kinases (CDKs) and their inhibitors (CDKIs).

Elevated expression of E6 and E7 have inhibitory effects on tumor suppressor proteins pRB and p53, which are responsible for removing the cells to an apoptotic pathway in response to DNA damage.

Cell regulatory protein pRB inhibits the cyclin-dependent kinase inhibitor gene p16 INK4a. When pRB is inactivated by E6 and E7, there is, increased expression of p16 INK4a.

Studies have shown that p16 INK4a is a specific biomarker to identify dysplastic cervical epithelium in the section of cervical biopsy samples and cervical smears.[65,66]

Chapter 16

Polarprobe (Polartechnics Ltd, Sydney, Australia)[67]

Polarprobe is a portable optoelectronic instrument that detects the existence of cervical cancer and precancer by measuring two sets of physical parameters: Voltage decay and the scattering of various wavelengths of light.

PRINCIPLE

1. When an electrical current is applied to a tissue, it causes the current to flow. The cell structure (cellular capacitance) and cell membrane and cellular fluid (conductance-resistance) attempt to prevent the decay of the applied voltage. The pattern of voltage decay over time varies with different types of tissues.
2. When light is focused on a tissue, depending on the character of the tissue, the light is transmitted and scattered at various wavelengths.

Polarprobe uses both these electrical and optical information and using a computer algorithm draws a statistical reference about the likelihood of malignancy.

The Polarprobe tip is 5 mm in diameter and 15 cm long. It has electrodes that come into contact with the tissue of the cervix. They polarize the tissue by applying a 1.2 V direct current source to the tissue, and the Polarprobe measures the pattern of electrical decay. The probe tip also has light-emitting diodes, each of which is pulsed at different wavelengths. The reflected light is read on a photoelectrode. The results are grouped into six tissue types.

Advantages

- Polarprobe provides instantaneous results.
- It is useful in developing countries with high-risk poor-compliant population where 'see and treat' approach can be utilized.

Chapter 17

Laser-induced Fluorescence[68]

Depending upon the chemical and morphological composition of individual tissues, low-powered laser illumination induces various endogenous tissue fluorescence. This spectroscopic difference, if detectable, can be used to differentiate normal from abnormal tissue. This technology is not available for widespread use, but may have a role to play in future.

Chapter 18

Speculoscopy

In speculoscopy, after applying acetic acid, the cervix is visualized under low-power magnification using specialized 'blue-white' chemiluminescent light. Depending upon the nature of the tissue examined, the intensity and distribution of the chemiluminescent light reflected from the tissue vary.

In this procedure, the inner aspect of the upper speculum blade contains peroxyoxate chemical, which gets activated to produce blue-white chemilumine-scent light. The cervix and vagina are washed with 3% to 5% acetic acid and inspected with magnifying 'loupes'. Any acetowhitening is considered positive. It relies on the presence of acetowhite epithelium without looking for atypical vessels.[69]

Chapter 19
Cervicography

In cervicography, after applying acetic acid to the cervix, using special cameras with macrolens, high-quality photographs of the cervix taken. These photographs are later interpreted by the experts in the field.

ADVANTAGES

- Less costly
- Photographs can be taken by paramedical personnel also.

LIMITATIONS

- It is a highly sensitive tool to evaluate the ectocervical transformation zone, but cannot evaluate the endocervical canal
- Therefore, it is most sensitive in young women in whom most of the TZ is ectocervical. As the woman ages and the TZ recede into the endocervical canal, cervix cannot be evaluated by cervicography.

Cervicography detects nearly all true high-grade lesions when the TZ is visible, but its sensitivity falls when the TZ recedes into the endocervical canal.[69]

Chapter 20

Colposcopy Training Log Book

A. INTRODUCTION

1. Purpose of the Log Book

The main purpose of the log book is to help you monitor your own competence. Its second purpose is to describe the minimum competence level expected of you at the end of your training.

2. Modules of the Curriculum

The log book has two main sections, the theoretical understanding and the practical one.

The *theoretical* understanding module is divided into five modules with a number of individual subjects. When you have addressed that topic in your reading and feel confident about it, then tick the relevant box.

The *practical* experience section is divided into seven separate modules. Each module contains a number of targets which require varying levels of competence to be attained during the course of your training.

3. Levels of Competence in Practical Experience Section

There are four levels of competence:
Level 1: Observe the activity being carried out.
Level 2: Carry out the whole activity under direct supervision
  The trainer is present throughout
Level 3: Carry out the procedure under indirect supervision
  The trainer need not be present but should be available to give opinion, to provide help and advice.
Level 4: Independent competence, no need for supervision

4. Number of Colposcopies to be Done

Cases to be observed	50
Cases to be managed under direct supervision	20
Cases to be managed under indirect supervision	20

B. THEORETICAL UNDERSTANDING

1. Normal Cervix

1.1 Normal structure
1.2 Metaplasia
1.3 The transformation zone
1.4 Changes with age
1.5 Tissue basis of colposcopic appearance
  – Role of epithelium
  – Role of stroma
  – Role of surface configuration

2. Equipment

2.1 The colposcope
2.2
  • Its parts
  • Filters
  • Magnifications
  • Focal length
2.3 Type of specula

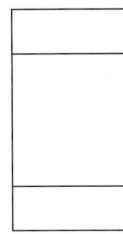

2.4 The role and use of saline and green filter
2.5 The role and use of acetic acid
2.6 The role and use of Lugol's iodine
2.7 The role and use of Monsel's solution
2.8 Principles of sterilization/decontamination of colposcopy clinic equipment

3. The Colposcopy Procedure

3.1 Use of saline and green filter
3.2 Use of acetic acid and interpretation of findings
3.3 Use of Lugol's iodine and interpretation of findings
4. **Understanding of Normal Colposcopic Findings**
5. **Understanding of Abnormal Colposcopic Findings**

C. PRACTICAL CONSIDERATIONS

1. Preliminary Skills

LEVEL 1 2 3 4

1.1 Take a relevant history
1.2 Position the patient
1.3 Pass a speculum
1.4 Perform bimanual examination
1.5 Perform a smear including use of endobrush

2. Colposcopic Examination

LEVEL 1 2 3 4

2.1 Identify the transformation zone (TZ)
2.2 Examine the TZ with saline and green filter
2.3 Examine the TZ with acetic acid
2.4 Examine the TZ with Lugol's iodine
2.5 Expose the endocervix with endocervical speculum
2.6 Recognize abnormal vascular patterns

3. Normal Cervix

LEVEL 1 2 3 4

3.1 Original squamous epithelium
3.2 Columnar epithelium
3.3 Metaplasia
3.4 Pregnancy
3.5 Postmenopausal cervix

4. Abnormal Lower Genital Tract

LEVEL 1 2 3 4

4.1 Low-grade cervical abnormality
4.2 High-grade cervical abnormality
4.3 Microinvasive carcinoma
4.4 Invasive carcinoma
4.5 VaIN
4.6 Determine the extent of abnormal epithelium
4.7 Recognize the infection
4.8 Recognize wart virus infection

5. Practical Procedures

LEVEL 1 2 3 4

5.1 Administration of local analgesia
5.2 Determine where to take directed biopsies
5.3 Directed cervical biopsy
5.4 Directed vaginal biopsy
5.5 Controlling of bleeding from the biopsy site
5.6 Performing endocervical curettage

6. Administration

LEVEL 1 2 3 4

6.1 Documentation of cervical findings
6.2 Arrange appropriate after-care/follow-up
6.3 Arrange referrals

7. Communication

LEVEL
1 2 3 4

7.1 Understand psychological effects of colposcopy

7.2 Able to counsel patients prior to colposcopy/treatment

7.3 Able to counsel patients after colposcopy/treatment

CASES MANAGED UNDER DIRECT SUPERVISION

No.	Date	Hosp.	IP No.	Smear	VIA/VILI	Colposcopy findings	Colposcopic impression

CASES MANAGED UNDER INDIRECT SUPERVISION

No.	Date	Hosp.	IP No.	Smear	VIA/VILI	Colposcopy findings

References

1. Ferlay J, Bray F, Pisani, et al. GLOBOCAN 2002: Cancer Incidence, Mortality and Prevalence Worldwide, IARC, Cancer Base No. 5, Version 2.0 (IARC Press;Lyon;2004).
2. World Health Organization (WHO). Regional Office for South-East Asia, Noncommunicable Diseases, South-East Asia Region: A profile. (New Delhi: WHO; 2002).
3. Miller AB. Cervical cancer screening programs: Managerial guidelines. WHO; Geneva: 1992.
4. Sankaranarayanan R, Budukh AM, Rajkumar R. Effective screening programmes for cervical cancer in low and middle income developing countries. Bulle: 2001;79(10).
5. Murthy NS, Agarwal SS, Prabhakar AK, Sharma S, Das DK. Estimation of reduction of lifetime risk of cervical cancer through one lifetime screening. Neoplasma. 1993;40(4):255-8.
6. Stjernsward J, et al. Plotting a new course for cervical cancer screening in developing countries: World Health Forum, 1987;8:42-5.
7. Frost JK, Gynecologic cytopathology. In: Gynecology (8th ed). Novak ER, Jones GS, Jones HW (Eds). The Baltimore Williams and Wilkins Company, 1971.
8. Hatch KD. Handbook of Colposcopy: Diagnosis and treatment of lower genital tract neoplasia and HPV infections. Boston, MA: Little Brown, 1989.
9. RL Giuntole and RE Briston, Cervical cancer. In: Danforth's Obstetrics & Gynecology, 10th. 2008, Lippincott Williams & Wilkins, Philadelphia. RS Gibbs, BY Karlan, AF Haney and I Nygaard.
10. Smith JS, Green J, Berrington dG, et al. Cervical cancer and use of hormonal contraceptives: a systematic review. Lancet 2003;361:1159-67.
11. Centres for Disease Control and Prevention. Sexually Transmitted Disease Guidelines. MMWR Morb Mortal wkly. 1993;42:90-100.
12. FX Bosch, YL Qiao, Castellsague X. The epidemiology of human papillomavirus infection and its association with cervical cancer. Int J Gynecol Obstet. 2006;94: supplement 1:S8-S21.
13. Castle PE, Hillier SL, Rabe LK, Hildesheim A, Herrero R, Bratti MC, et al. An association of cervical inflammation with High-grade Cervical Neoplasia in women infected with Oncogenic Human Papillomavirus (HPV). Cancer Epidemiology, Biomarkers and Prevention. 2001;10:1021-7.
14. Ames BN, Gold IS and Willett WC. The causes and prevention of cancer. Proc. Natl Acad. Sci. USA 1995;92:5258-65.
15. Munoz N, Bosch Fx, de Sanjose S, et al. Epidemiologic classification of HPV types associated with cervical cancer. N Eng J Med. 2003;348:518-27.
16. Frazer IH. Prevention of cervical cancer through Papilloma virus vaccination. Nat Rev Immunol. 2004;4:46-54.
17. Snijders PJ, Steenbergen RD, Heideman DA, Meijer CJ. HPV-mediated cervical carcinogenesis: Concepts and clinical implications. J Pathol. 2006; 208(2):152-64.
18. Melkert PW, Hopman E, van den Brule AJ, et al. Prevalence of HPV in cytomorphologically normal cervical smears, as determined by the polymerase chain reaction, is age-dependent. Int J Cancer. 1993;53:919-23.
19. Wallin KL, Wiklund F, Angstrom J, Bergman F, et al. Type-specific persistence of human papilloma virus DNA before the development of invasive cervical carcinoma. N Eng J Med. 1999;341:1633-8.
20. Preventing cervical cancer in Low-resource settings: from research to practice, Conference Report. Thailand, Dec. 2005, Sanghvi S, Lacoste M, McCormick M (Eds). JHPIEGO, Baltimore, Maryland.
21. Ostor AG. Natural history of cervical intraepithelial Neoplasia: a critical review. Int J Gynecol Pathol. 1993;12:186-92.
22. Winer RL, Kiviat NB, Hughes JP, et al. Development and duration of human papillomavirus lesions, after initial infection. J Infect Dis. 2005;191(5):731-8.
23. Wright TC, COX JT, Massad LS, et al. The 2001 consensus guidelines for the management of women with cervical cytological abnormality. JAMA. 2002;287:2120-9.
24. Germain M, Heaton R, Erickson D, et al. A comparison of the three most common Papanicolaou smear collection techniques. Obstet Gynecol. 1994;84:168-73.

25. Harer WB, Valenzuela G Jr, Lebo D. Lubrication of the vaginal introitus and speculum does not affect Papanicolaou smears. Obstet Gynecol. 2002;100:887-8.
26. Michael TF, Irwig L, Macaskill P. Meta-analysis of Pap test Accuracy. Am J Epidemiol. 1995;141(7):680-9.
27. Evidence Report/Technology Assessment, Number 5. Evaluation of cervical cytology. Maryland, AHCPR Publication No. 99-E010, February 1999.
28. Nanda K, Mc Crory DC, Myers ER, Bastian LA, Hasselblad V, Jason D. Hickey, et al. Matchar. Accuracy of the Papanicolaou Test in screening for, and follow-up of, cervical cytologic abnormalities: A Systematic review. Ann Intern Med. 2000;132:810-19.
29. Nuovo HM, Melnikov J, Howell LP. New tests for cervical cancer screening. Am Fam Physician. 2001;64:780-6.
30. Duggan MA. Papnet-assisted primary screening of cervico-vaginal smears, Eur J Gynaecol Oncol. 2000;21:35-42.
31. Ouwerkerk-Noordam E, Boon ME, Beck S. Computer-assisted primary screening of cervical smears using the PAPNET method: Comparison with conventional screening and evaluation of the role of the cytologist. Cytopathology. 1994; 5: 211-18.
32. Wilbur DC, Prey MU, Miller WM. The Auto Pap system for primary screening in cervical cytology. Comparing the results of a prospective, intended use study with routine manual practice. Acta Cytol. 1998; 42:214-220.
33. Ronco G, Cuzick J, Pierotti P, et al. Accuracy of liquid-based versus conventional cytology: overall results of new technologies for cervical cancer screening: randomized controlled trial. BMJ. 2007 (7); 335(7609):28. Epub. 2007, May 21.
34. Davey E, d' Assuncao J, Irvvig L, Macaskill P, Chan SF, Richards A, et al. Accuracy of reading liquid-based cytology slides using the Thin Prep Imager compared with conventional cytology: prospective study. BMJ. 2007;335 (7609):31.
35. Sasieni P, Adams J, Cuzick J. Benefits of cervical screening at different ages: Evidence from the UK Audit of screening histories. Br J Cancer. 2003;89:88-93.
36. Saslow D, Runowicz CD, Solomon D, et.al. American Cancer Society guideline for the early detection of cervical Neoplasia and cancer. Cancer J Clin. 2002;52:342-62.
37. Melkert PW, Hopman E, van den Brule AJ, et al. Prevalence of HPV in cytomorphologically normal cervical smears, as determined by the polymerase chain reaction, is age-dependent. Int J Cancer. 1993;53:919-23.
38. Villa LL, Lynette Denny, Methods for detection of HPV infection and its clinical utility. Int J Gynecol Obstet. 2006; 94:571-580.
39. Manos MM, Kinney WK, Hurley LB, Sherman ME, Shieh Ngai J, Kurman RJ, et al. Identifying women with cervical neoplasia using human papillomavirus testing for equivocal Papanicolaou results: JAMA. 1999;281:1605-10.
40. The Atypical squamous cells of undetermined significance/low-grade squamous intraepithelial lesion; Triage study (ALTS) Group. Human Papilloma virus testing for triage of women with cytologic evidence of low-grade squamous intraepithelial lesion: baseline data from a randomized trial. J Nati. Cancer Inst. 2000; 92(5);397-402.
41. Paraskevaidis E, Arbyn M, Sotiriadis A, et al. The role of HPV DNA testing in the follow-up period after treatment for CIN: a systematic review of the literature. Cancer Treat Rev. 2004; 30: 205-211.
42. American College of Obstetricians and Gynecologists. Cervical cytology screening, ACOG. Practice Bulletin. Number 45, August 2003. Int J Gynecol. Obstet. 2003;83:237-47.
43. Lorincz AT, Richart RM. Human papillomavirus DNA testing as an adjunct to cytology in cervical screening programs. Arch Pathol Lab Med. 2003;127:959-68.
44. Iftner T, Villa LL, Human Papillomavirus technologies. J Nat. Cancer Inst. Mono. 2003;31:80-8.
45. Stoler MH, Schiffman M. Interobserver reproducibility of cervical cytologic and histologic interpretations: realistic estimates from the ASCUS-LSIL Triage study. JAMA 2001; 285;1500-5.
46. Boardman LA, Kennedy CM. Management of atypical squamous cells, Low-grade squamous intraepithelial lesions, and cervical intraepithelial neoplasia. Obstetrics and Gynecology. 2008;35(4):599-614.
47. Jones BA, Novis DA. Follow-up of abnormal gynecologic cytology: a college of American pathologists Q-Probes study of 16,132 cases from 306 laboratories. Arch Pathol Lab Med. 2000;124:665-7.
48. Results of randomized trial on the management of cytology interpretations of atypical squamous cells of undetermined significance. ASCUS-LSIL Triage study (ALTS) group. Am J obstet Gynecol. 2003;188:1383-92.
49. Schiffman M, Adrianza ME. ASCUS-LSIL triage study: design, methods and characteristics of trial participants. Acta Cytol. 2000;44:726-42.
50. Insinga RP, Glass AG, Rush BB. Diagnoses and outcomes in cervical cancer screening: a population-based study. Am J Obstet Gynecol. 2004;191:105-13.
51. Sherman ME, Castle PE, Solomon D. Cervical cytology of atypical squamous cells—Cannot exclude high-grade squamous intraepithelial lesions (ASC-H): Characteristics and histologic outcomes. Cancer. 2006;108:298-305.
52. Dunn TS, Burke M, Shwayder J. A "see and treat" management for high-grade squamous intraepithelial lesion pap smears. J Low Genit Tract Dis. 2003;7:104-6.
53. Jones BA, Davey DD. Quality management in gynaecologic cytology using interlaboratory comparison. Arch Pathol Lab Med. 2000;124: 672-8.
54. Sharpless KE, Schnatz PF, Mandavilli S, Greene JF, Sorosky J. Dysplasia associated with atypical glandular cells on cervical cytology. Obstet Gynecol. 2005;105; 494-500.
55. Schnatz PF, Guile M, O' Sullivan DM, et al. Clinical significance of atypical glandular cells on cervical cytology. Obstet Gynecol. 2006;107(3):70-8.
56. Siebers AG, Verbeek AL, Massuer LF, et al. Normal appearing endometrial cells in cervical smears of asymptomatic postmenopausal women have predictive value for significant endometrial pathology. Int J Gynecol Cancer. 2006;16:1069-74.
57. Coppleson M, Pixley E, Reid B: The tissue basis of colposcopic appearances. In colposcopy: A scientific and practical approach to the cervix, vagina and vulva in health and disease (3rd ed). Springfield, IL, Charles C Thomas. 1986; p. 114.

58. Reid R, Scalz P. Genital warts and cervical cancer. VII. An improved colposcopic index for differentiating benign papilloma viral infections from high-grade cervical intraepithelium neoplasia. Am J Obstet Gynecol. 1985;153; 611-8.
59. Greenberg, MD. Reid's Colposcopic Index. In Colposcopy Principles and Practice. An Integrated Textbook and Atlas, Apgar BS, Brotzman GL and Spitzer M (Eds), WB Saunders Company, Philadelphia, USA, 2002.
60. Kavita NS, Chakma T, Verma S, Sharma D, Khare S. Colposcopic assessment of the cervix using the simplified Reid's Colposcopic Index Method. Current Science. 2009;96 (3):386-91.
61. International Agency for Research on Cancer (IARC). Handbooks of cancer prevention. Vol 10: Cervix cancer screening. IARC: France. 2005.
62. Sankaranarayanan R, Wesley R, Thara S, Dhakad N, Chandralekha B, Sebastian P, et al. Test characteristics of visual inspection with 4% acetic acid (VIA) and Lugol's iodine (VILI) in cervical cancer screening in Kerala, India. Int J Cancer. 2003;106(3):404-8.
63. Legood R, Gray AM, Mahe C, Wolstenholme J, Jayant K, Nene BM, et al. Screening of cervical cancer in India: How much will it cost? A trial-based analysis of the cost per case detected. Int J Cancer. 2005;117(6):981-7.
64. Sankara Narayanan R, Basu P, Wesley RS, Mahe C, Keita N, Mbalawa CC, et al. IARC Multicentric study group on cervical cancer early detection. Accuracy of visual screening for cervical neoplasia: Results from an IARC multicentric study in India and Africa. Int J Cancer. 2004;110(6):907-13.
65. Abeer A Bahnassy, Abdel Rahman N Zekri, Maha Saleh, Mohammad Lotayef, Manar Moneir, Osama Shawki. The possible role of cell cycle regulators in multistep process of HPV-associated cervical carcinoma. BMC Clinical Pathology. 2007;7:4
66. Klaes R, Friedrich T, Spitovsky D, Ridder R, et al. Overexpression of p. 16 INK4A as a specific marker for dysplastic and neoplastic epithelial cells of the cervix uteri. Int J Cancer. 2001;92(2):276-84.
67. Quek SC, Mould T, Canfell K, et al. The Polarprobe-emerging technology for cervical cancer screening. Singapore. Ann Acad Med. 1998;27: p. 717
68. Lam S, Hung J, Kennedy S, et al. Detection of dysplasia and carcinoma in situ by radiofluorometry. Am Rev Resp Dis. 1992; 146:1458-66.
69. Spitzer M. Cervical screening adjuncts. Recent advances. Am J Obstet Gynecol. 1998;179(2):544-56.

Index

Page numbers followed by *t* refer to table and *f* refer to figure

A

Acetic acid
　on cervical epithelium, effect of 47
　visual inspection with 89, 90
Acetowhite epithelium 53, 56
Acetowhite reaction 67
Acquired immunodeficiency syndrome 9
Adenocarcinoma 17, 22, 41, 61
　in situ 16, 18*f*, 22, 41
American Cancer Society 28
American College of Obstetricians and Gynecologists 28
American Society for Colposcopy and Cervical Pathology 21
Atrophy 53
Atypical glandular cells, management of 41, 41*f*, 42*f*
Atypical squamous cell, management of 37
Automated cervical screening technique 20

B

Blood vessels, nature of 67

C

Cancer 94
　prevention 2
Carcinoma
　adenosquamous 17
　cervical 8, 8*f*, 9, 10
　endometrial 42
　epidermoid 17
　invasive 95
Cells
　cycle markers 96
　endocervical 22
　endometrial 22
Cervical adenocarcinoma, cytology of 34
Cervical cancer
　natural history of 14
　prevention, alliance for 89
Cervical carcinoma
　cause of 8
　pathogenesis of 12
　screening tests for 20
Cervical cytology
　cervical 20
　reporting of 21*t*
　sample collection for 22
Cervical epithelium, natural history of 51
Cervical intraepithelial neoplasia, histology of 15
Cervicography 20, 100
Cervix
　adenocarcinoma of 19*f*
　carcinoma of 19*f*
　ectropion of 75, 75*f*
　external os of 67*f*
　in pregnancy, ectopy of 3*f*
　infection of 77
　large ectropion of 75*f*
　low-grade lesion in anterior lip of 83*f*
　portio vaginalis of 81*f*
　postmenopausal 3*f*, 4*f*, 57*f*, 63*f*, 80*f*
　squamous cell carcinoma of 18*f*, 199*f*
Chlamydia trachomatis 26
CIN lesions
　different grades of 18*f*
　natural history of 14*t*
Clear cell adenocarcinomas 17
Colposcope 44, 45*f*
Colposcopic findings
　abnormal 53, 56
　documentation of 66
　normal 53, 54
Colposcopy 43
　appearance 76
　camera for 44
　equipment 44
　in invasive cancer 86
　in pregnancy 77
　indications for 43
　method 44
　of adolescence 55
　procedure 102
　satisfactory 65, 65*f*
　technique of 49
　training log book 101
　unsatisfactory 53, 65, 66
Columnar epithelium 4, 53, 93
Condylomas 94
Contraception, method of 48
Coppleson's grading of colposcopic findings 67
Curettage, endocervical 39, 44, 49
Cusco's speculum 22, 49, 81*f*
Cytoplasm 5

D

Digital video colposcopy 45
Döderlein's bacillus 6

E

Ectocervical biopsy 49
Embryonal rhabdomyosarcoma 17
Endocervical assessment, indications for 64
Endocervical brush, use of 24
Endocervical cells, normal 32*f*
Epithelial cell abnormalities 22
Epithelium 53
Exophytic condyloma 53

G

Glands, endocervical 5*f*
Glandular cells 22

H

High-grade squamous intraepithelial lesion 22, 34, 43
　management of 40
HPV
　DNA testing 29, 30
　　limitations of 31
　in cervix, lifecycle of 11*f*
　infection 12
　　diagnosis of 31
　　phases of 12*f*
　testing 20
　oncogenesis of 10
Human papillomavirus 8, 9*f*, 10
Hyperchromasia 15

I

Immature metaplastic squamous epithelium, tongues of 58f
Infection, evidence of 48
Inflammatory smears 33f
International Federation of Cervical Pathology and Colposcopy 53
Intraepithelial neoplasia, cervical 8, 20
Invasive cancers, histopathology of 17
Iodine staining 67, 72

K

Kogan's endocervical speculum 66, 66f

L

Large exophytic condyloma 84f
Laser induced fluorescence 20, 98
Leiomyosarcoma 17
Leukoplakia 53, 61, 63f, 95
Liquid-based thin-layer cytology 25
Lower genital tract, abnormal 102
Low-grade intraepithelial neoplasia 82
Low-grade squamous intraepithelial lesion 22
    cytology of 33
Lugol's iodine 67, 95
    application 92, 93f
    on cervical epithelium, effect of 48
    solution 44, 46, 68t
    visual inspection with 2, 89, 91

M

Melanomas 17
Metaplasia 8, 95
    colposcopic appearance of 75
Metaplastic epithelium 6, 56f, 64f
    vascular pattern of 55
Metaplastic squamous epithelium 6f, 76f
Mixed Müllerian tumor 17
Modified Reid colposcopic index 68t
Molecular biology techniques 31
Monsel's paste 44, 50
Monsel's solution 46
Multiple Nabothian cysts 79f

N

Nabothian cyst 5f, 7, 75f, 78f, 79f
Neisseria gonorrhoea 26
Noncorrelating colposcopy, clarification of 30
Normal and abnormal cells of cervix, cytology of 32

O

Original columnar epithelium 54
Original squamocolumnar junction 51
Original squamous epithelium 53, 54

P

Pap smear testing, frequency of 27
Papanicolaou smear 20, 49
Papilloma virus
    infection, subclinical 43, 67
    phylogenetic tree 9f
Parabasal cell atrophy 6
Petechial hemorrhages 4f
Plastic broom, use of 24
Polymerase chain reaction 31
Polyp, endocervical 5f, 75, 79f
Post-hysterectomy smear 28
Postmenopausal period 6

R

RCI, advantages of 74
Reid's colposcopic assessment system 67
Ring or sponge forceps 44

S

Sarcoma botyroids 17
Schiller's test 29, 48, 61, 92
Sexually transmitted infectious 9
Silver nitrate sticks 44, 46, 47
Simplified Reid's colposcopic index 74f
Speculoscopy 20, 99
Speculum, endocervical 44f
Squamocolumnar junction 4, 6, 51f
Squamous and columnar epithelium 54f
Squamous cell 22
    atypical 22, 33, 37, 41
    carcinoma 17, 22
        cytology of 34
Squamous epithelium 4, 5f
    of normal cervix 4f
Squamous metaplasia 51f, 52
    tongues of 52f
Strawberry cervix 77
Stroma 53

T

Tissues, colposcopic appearance of 53
Trichomonas vaginalis 21, 93
Tumors
    carcinoid 17
    epithelial 17
    neuroendocrine 17
    nonepithelial 17
TZ with Ayre's spatula, sampling of 23f

U

Ulcer 53

V

Vessels, atypical 53, 59, 72f
VIA and VILI, technique of 91
Video colposcope 46f
Visual inspection methods 89
Visual screening 89
    techniques 89

Z

Zoom focus knobs 45